ELEVATED EVERYDAY PALEO

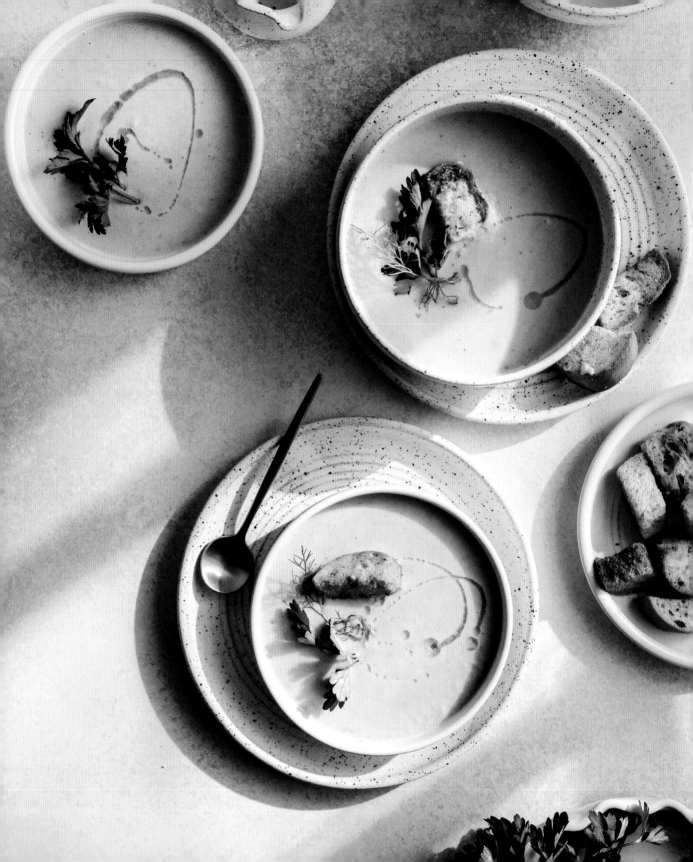

ELEVATED EVERYDAY PALEO

60 SIMPLE-MADE-SPECIAL RECIPES FOR HEALTHY EVERYDAY COOKING

MORIAH SAWTELLE

PAGE STREET
PUBLISHING CO.

PAGE STREET
PUBLISHING CO.

Copyright © 2022 Moriah Sawtelle

First published in 2022 by
Page Street Publishing Co.
27 Congress Street, Suite 1511
Salem, MA 01970
www.pagestreetpublishing.com

Distributed by Macmillan, sales in Canada by The Canadian Manda Group.

26   25   24   23   22   1   2   3   4   5

ISBN-13: 978-1-64567-492-4
ISBN-10: 1-64567-492-4

Library of Congress Control Number: 2021937889

Cover and book design by Moriah Sawtelle
Photography by Moriah Sawtelle

Printed and bound in the United States

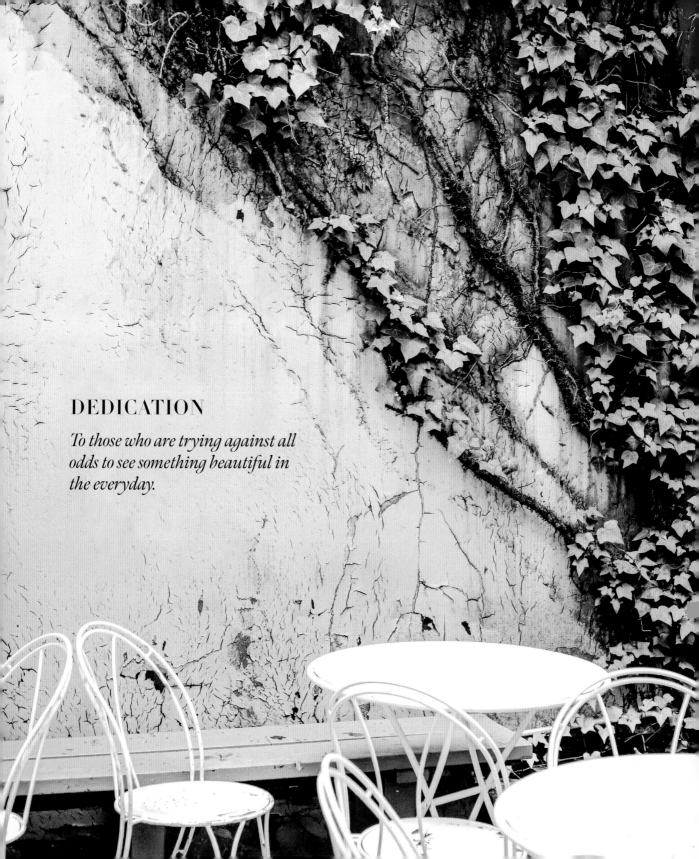

DEDICATION

To those who are trying against all odds to see something beautiful in the everyday.

CONTENTS

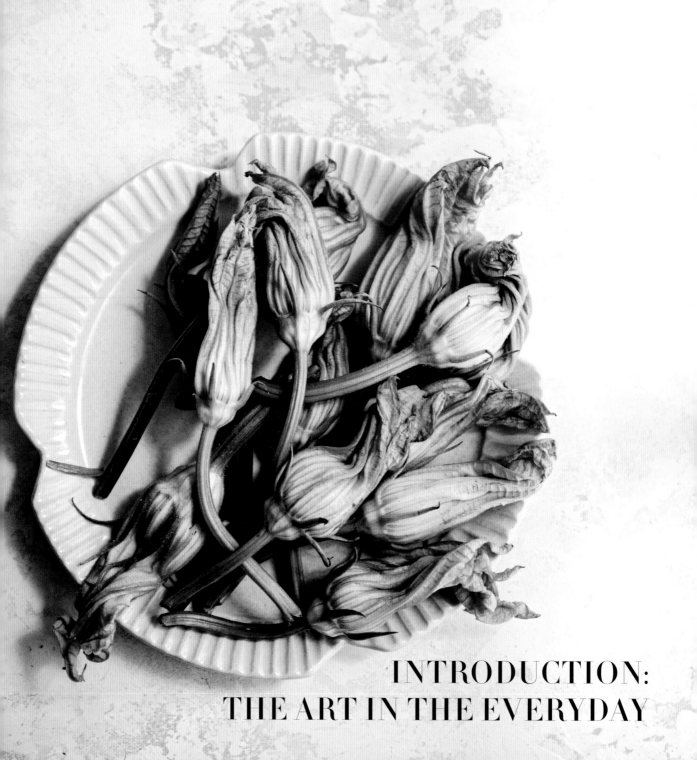

INTRODUCTION:
THE ART IN THE EVERYDAY

Life is sometimes hard. Things go wrong, in life and in love and in business and in friendship and in health and in all the other ways that life can go wrong.

And when things get tough, this is what you should do.

Make good art.

- NEIL GAIMAN

For me, creating has always been about optimism. It's a chance to look at broken pieces, an everyday task, or a challenging problem and say, "I can choose to see potential and make this beautiful."

This mentality has trickled down through the ventures I've taken on throughout my career, from building my creative agency and writing my blog to making this book. It's always been an optimistic scraping together of what I could find and tending to the pieces until I made something from the rubble.

It all started back as a teenager when I found I had celiac disease and a slew of other autoimmune symptoms that have followed me like a shadow into adulthood. Cooking for my numerous dietary restrictions was always a daunting, difficult thing that I preferred to avoid. Eating was, too. It was always followed by consequences. When I was twenty-one I realized my health had gotten away from me, and I could no longer avoid cooking and eating forever. I needed to heal, and it would come through whole-food ingredients and patience.

I started creating recipes and photographing them to share. The photography was fun, and sharing what I created was the only way I stayed motivated to keep at it. And the more I did it, the more I really, really loved the photography. My bad images slowly got better, and so did the recipes. And then I was shooting in restaurants and working with chefs—and this shadow that had loomed over me was now turning into art in the palms of my hands as I peeled carrots, picked herbs and pressed the shutter.

Now, food is my friend. It's helped me heal and given me the energy to build a life and business that I love. Cooking is my friend, too. I'm no Martha or Ina, and I still try to cook as little as possible if I'm being honest, but I love the process of looking at raw ingredients and the everyday task of making a meal and *making art with it.*

Maybe that's you. Maybe you don't inherently love cooking or you've had your own harrowing journey dealing with health issues and coming to terms with using food as medicine. Or maybe you just love putting a simple-yet-beautiful dish down on the table on a Monday night and feeling like in the midst of the mundane you found a moment of something special. This book is for you: a seat at the table for anyone who is trying against all odds to make something beautiful in the everyday. The art is always there. You just need to find it, piece it together and plate it.

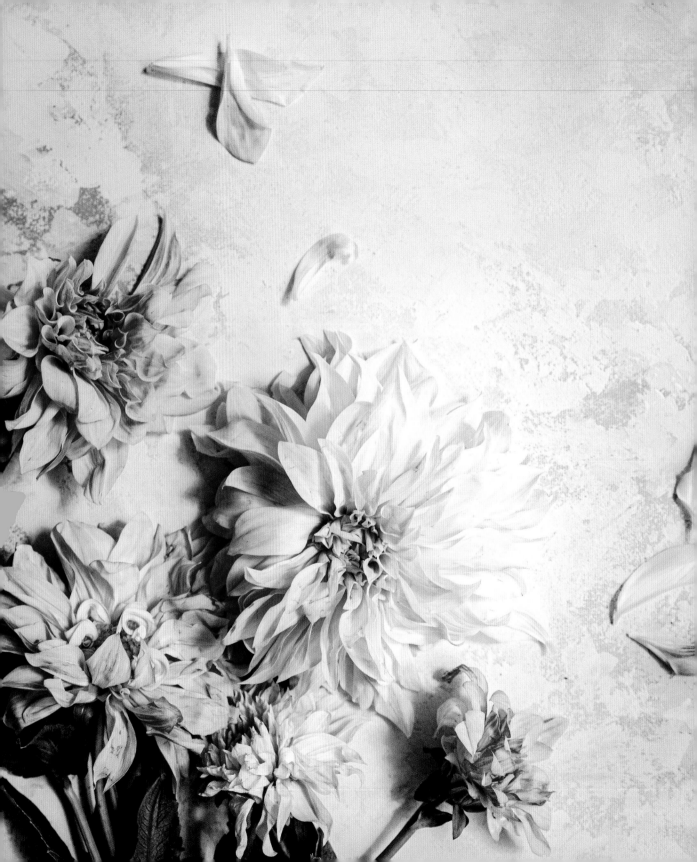

FOOD PHILOSOPHY

I want to take a moment to clarify that this isn't meant to be a diet book. In fact, this book isn't even trying to make you convert to Paleo. I myself don't eat one hundred percent Paleo. Rather, this is a book to help those on a limited diet, or those simply seeking health, to find some renewed joy in the kitchen.

My hope is that the word "Paleo" acts as a bit of a lighthouse, helping you to know that a bunch of whole-foods recipes are here for you to enjoy. But I also hope that you're able to take these recipes with their notes and suggestions and make them into your very own small victories scattered throughout the day, no matter what a healthy diet looks like for you.

In a sea of cookbooks, fad diets and confusing research, it can be incredibly overwhelming to decide what is truly the best way to eat for your own health. I've been on this roller coaster since I was thirteen, listening to far too many voices and cutting out too many foods. I was often doing more harm than good as I tried everything I could to tackle my health issues and finally feel like I had the energy to be a normal teenager and then twenty-something.

I'll spare you the nitty gritty, but from age thirteen to twenty-four I went on just about every autoimmune diet and health fad you can imagine. Food saved me when medicine couldn't, but the dogma of it all really broke me physically and psychologically before things got better. It seemed for years like my body wanted nothing to do with food, and nothing worked for me until I said "screw it" and decided to listen to what made sense for me and my own body. There is no diet name for what this is. It's just real food and real life, and a concerted effort to be aware of stressors outside of food that can mess with my digestion.

It would be hypocritical for me to tell you what to eat after the war I've fought in my own mind all of these years, but I can tell you this one rule that I've come to believe sums everything up: Food is about balance, nourishment and individuality.

So where does Paleo fit in, then? For me, Paleo best describes the baseline I return to when my autoimmune symptoms creep in. It's also a way of finding products or recipes that I know will be made of the ingredients I know to be beneficial: meat, vegetables, fruit, starches and healthy fats.

These recipes are the result of learning how to feed my body well. I love this crazy, wild, beautiful life so much that I've made a concerted effort over the past couple of years to make amends with this "chore." And I wanted to do it in a way that made something good from the hard years. I hope that you will also find food, and the kitchen, to be a welcome part of your life that gives you the energy to be and do your best.

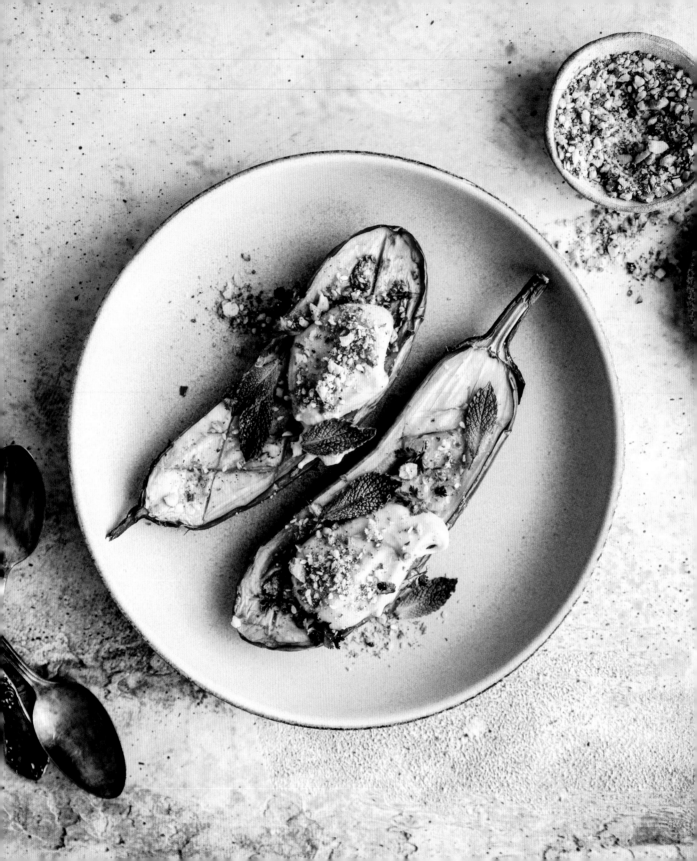

BEFORE YOU BEGIN

Cooking Gluten-Free and Grain-Free

If you're new to cooking gluten-free and grain-free, be patient. Mistakes are the unspoken ingredient in most recipes, especially when you are new to this process. Embrace the challenging recipes and turn to the easier ones when you need a quick win. Let yourself lean into this rewarding process.

A Sense of Place

My writing and recipes always come from imagining a sense of place: it adds an adventure and an extra layer of excitement to cooking. Most of these recipes are inspired by the crackling energy of New York City and the vast downtown food scene that has formed my career, though some call back to my New England roots or tan-lined days in Europe. Maybe it's just me romanticizing this entire thing, but I think it's extra fun to let these recipes whisk you away to their roots, so I've added in brief stories of how I learned about these flavors and ingredients.

Ingredients and Substitutions

Don't worry, I'm not into recipes that require you to do a pantry overhaul and hunt down a list of complicated ingredients. In fact, my pantry is one tiny shelf of items in my apartment, and that's all you should need to cook your way through this book.

Having good, quality ingredients is half of the battle—whether you're cooking gluten-free or not. Here, I'll fill you in on the items I turn to on a regular basis, so you can stock your own small-but-mighty pantry army and dive into the recipes.

Bone Broth

Mineral-rich bone broth is my liquid of choice for all of the soups and stews in this book. It's been a key component of my wellness journey, and it's something I use in my diet on a weekly basis to maintain my gut and overall health. I use Springbone Kitchen broth, which is a major bonus of living in New York City. If you're looking for another brand, you'll want to find something that is gelatinous when cold.

Cassava Flour

All of the baking in this book is done with my favorite grain-free flour: cassava. I use Bob's Red Mill, Thrive Market or Otto's, which I find to be comparable. To achieve a similar outcome, I recommend measuring by weight no matter what brand you're using. I've found the typical cup of cassava flour to weigh 130 grams, but I've found brands that are anywhere from 90 to 150 grams. So, it's really worth it to weigh your flours!

Cheese

My personal health journey has led me to a place where I believe that whole dairy sources are beneficial, so cheese is included in several recipes in this book. That said, it is always as a garnish and never essential to the flavor or integrity of a recipe. You can easily omit the cheese or use a plant-based cheese, if desired.

Chocolate

Good chocolate is *always* worth the money. Raaka is my absolute favorite brand. Bonus: They're Brooklyn based! I use their bars or baking chocolate in any recipe with chocolate in it. If you need an alternative, look for something made with real cocoa beans. Quality chocolate like Raaka is often naturally gluten- and dairy-free.

Eggs

I try to use pasture-raised eggs whenever I can—most notably in the breakfast recipes where the rich yolk and added health benefits can truly be appreciated. I always use room-temperature eggs when baking.

Milk

All of the recipes in this book that include milk use canned coconut milk. I always aim to use a brand that doesn't include any thickeners; coconut and water should be the only ingredients. Cows' dairy is the best substitution if you prefer to use another milk; almond milk could also be used if necessary. No matter what kind of milk I am using, I always make sure it is room temperature when baking.

Oil

I aim to use coconut oil, butter or ghee in most of my cooking because they are the most stable, saturated oils. I'll occasionally use high-quality olive oil for its flavor or when I want a liquid oil. If you need to substitute another oil, use one with a similar melting point as the one in the recipe.

Rice

After many years eating strict-Paleo, I realized that somewhere along the way I'd stopped listening to my body and followed a set of rules somewhat blindly. I've found that my body actually responds well to rice, and I *enjoy* it, which is an important component when finding what foods are right for you. I love serving curry or a stir-fry over rice. If that isn't your thing, cauliflower rice works nicely, too!

Cookware

My kitchen space is about forty square feet, so having a few reliable, versatile, high-quality pans and utensils is super important. I've relied on Material Kitchen for my knives, pans, cutting boards and utensils for a few years now, and I've never looked back. They fit perfectly in my tiny kitchen and get the job done every time.

Salt

I put Maldon salt on everything I consume, even in juice. It's a mineral-rich salt that adds depth of flavor while also helping your body to get enough of the minerals that most of us are deficient in. If you don't have access to Maldon, I'd recommend grabbing another high-quality flakey salt, such as Redmond Real Salt or Jacobsen Salt, to finish your recipes.

Storage

Perishable, gluten-free foods don't keep as long as their glutenous counterparts. Most recipes will keep for 5 days in an airtight container in the fridge.

Sweeteners

Organic cane sugar is my go-to granulated sweetener for baking. Coconut sugar can also be substituted 1:1. I typically lean on maple syrup and honey for liquid sweeteners; they can be used interchangeably depending on what you have on hand.

Tahini

Tahini appears in this book many, many times. It's a staple in my cooking and one of my favorite flavor additions to dips or vegetable dishes. I am a die-hard fan of Seed + Mill, which is the smoothest, creamiest tahini I've found yet. It's perfect for baking and gives consistently good results every time.

Other Substitutions

Even if you think you don't, you have the intuition that can help you figure out substitutions when cooking. You'll grow more confident with more practice, but experiment with what sounds good and what you have available. If you're still getting acquainted with this whole "cooking" thing, while you learn flavors try to sub within categories (e.g., starches, meats, vegetables) for best results.

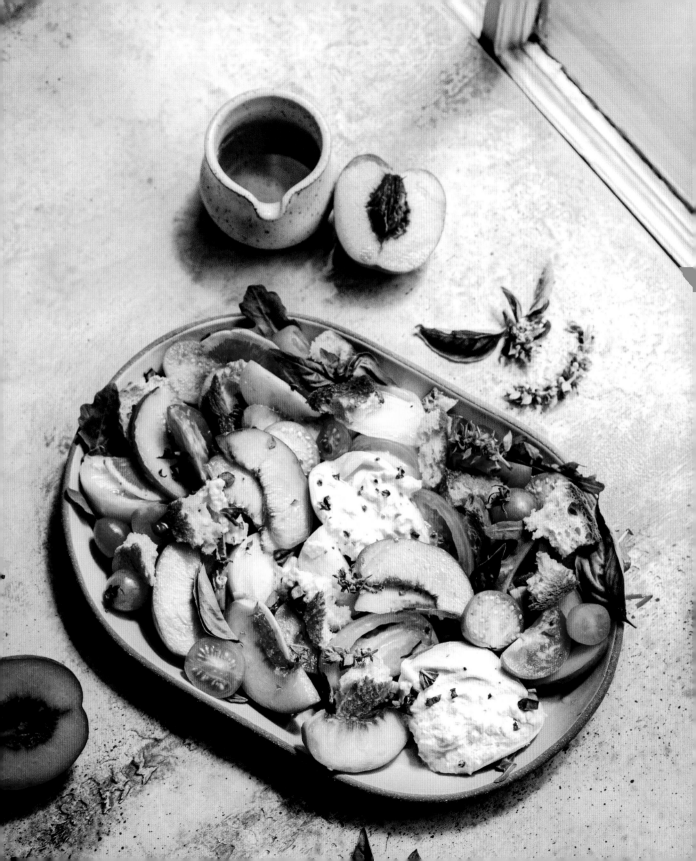

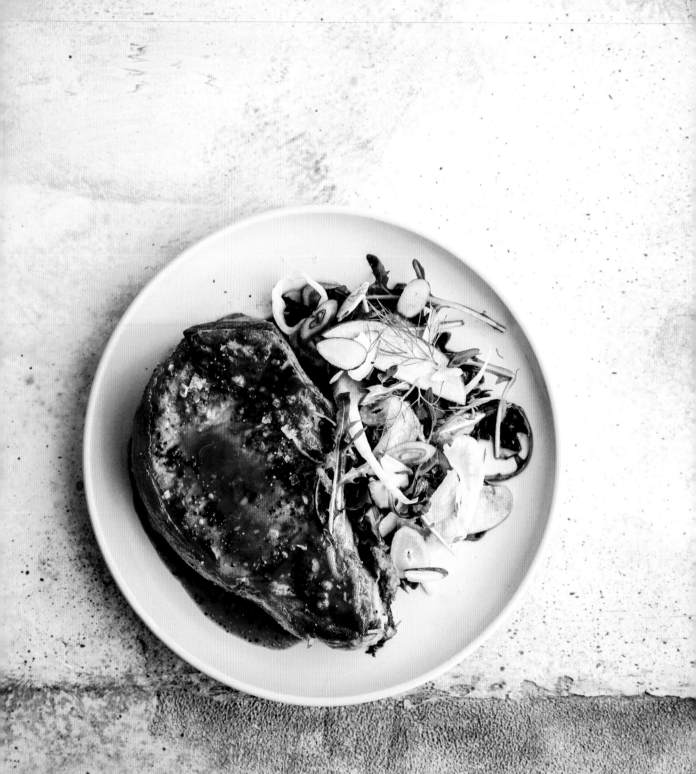

Maybe it's not about having a beautiful day,
but about finding beautiful moments.

—ANNA WHITE, *MENDED*

ELEVATED DINNERS

It's important for you to know that what I do, anyone can do. These meals aren't productions. They're just what I aim for on a good day—a day where I'm better at finding the beauty in the texture of life. It's about celebrating and elevating the in-between moments, which are often meals. Though I'm also very guilty of cracking two eggs in a pan and eating them on the couch in my best baggy sweatpants, because that's life.

I think there's something about the process of creating a nourishing meal with your hands that feels therapeutic, whether it's something comforting like Cranberry-Balsamic Short Ribs (page 19), or a fresh and vibrant dish, like my Arctic Char with Lemon Salsa Verde and Grapefruit (page 27). Maybe it's a cheap thrill, but making beauty from small things makes life more interesting and more inviting. It's all what you make of it. And in this book, we're making it delicious.

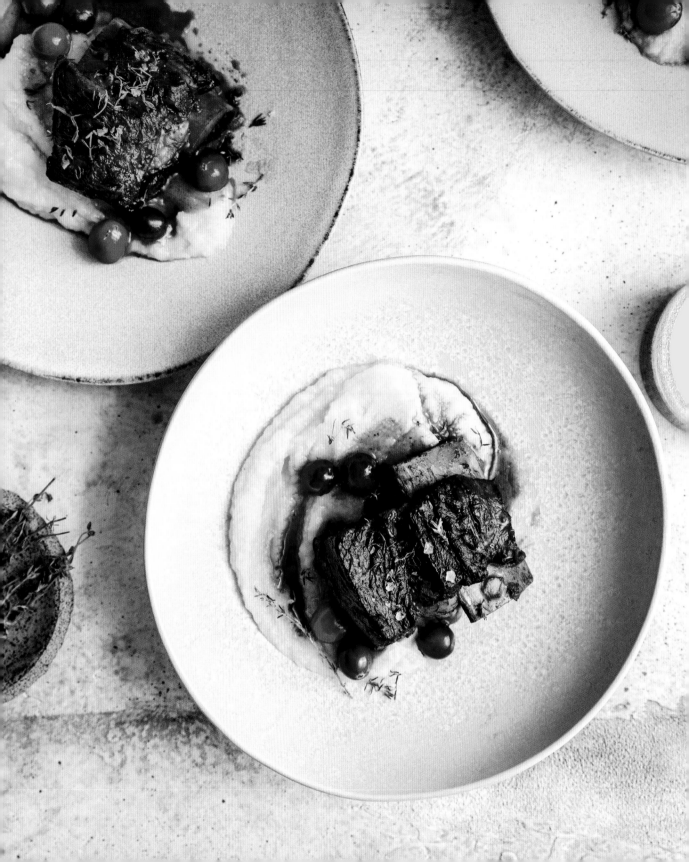

CRANBERRY-BALSAMIC SHORT RIBS

Nothing livens up a monochromatic winter like a dish with cranberries. And nothing brings out the flavor of cranberries like balsamic vinegar and red wine. It's the perfect sweet-and-tangy sauce for braising beef short ribs, and the result is pure melt-in-your-mouth goodness. There is something comforting and indulgent about this flavor combo that I can't quite articulate, but I do know this: this is the kind of food you serve to those you love deeply.

Serves: 4

FOR THE SHORT RIBS

3–4 lbs (1.4–1.8 kg) beef short ribs, cut into 2- to 3-inch (5- to 8-cm) pieces

½ tsp sea salt

½ tsp black pepper

2 tbsp (30 ml) olive oil

4 cloves garlic, minced

2 shallots, sliced

1 cup (240 ml) red wine

¼ cup (60 ml) balsamic vinegar

2½ cups (600 ml) beef bone broth

1 tbsp (2 g) fresh thyme, plus more for garnish

1½ cups (150 g) fresh cranberries

FOR THE PARSNIP MASH

5 large parsnips (600 g), peeled and roughly chopped

2 cloves garlic, minced

2 tbsp (30 ml) olive oil

⅓ cup (80 ml) milk of choice

½ tsp sea salt, plus more to taste

¼ tsp black pepper, plus more to taste

Preheat the oven to 325°F (163°C).

To make the short ribs: Season the short ribs with the salt and pepper. Heat the oil in a large Dutch oven over medium-high heat and brown the ribs for 3 minutes on each side. Remove the seared ribs to a plate and set aside.

Add the garlic and shallots to the pot. Sauté, stirring frequently, for 2 to 3 minutes, or until the garlic is aromatic and the shallots have softened. Deglaze with the red wine, then stir in the vinegar, broth and thyme. Return the ribs to the pot, then add the cranberries. Cover the pot and place it in the oven for 2½ to 3 hours, until the ribs are tender and falling off the bone.

While the ribs cook, make the parsnip mash: Place the parsnips in a large saucepan with enough water to cover by 1 inch (2.5 cm). Bring the water to a boil and cook for 15 minutes, or until the parsnips are fork-tender. Drain the parsnips and place them in a food processor fitted with an S-blade. Add the garlic, olive oil, milk, salt and pepper. Blend until the parsnips are smooth and creamy. Add more salt and pepper to taste, if needed.

Serve the short ribs over the mashed parsnips with drippings from the pot and a garnish of fresh thyme.

CHILI-RUBBED SALMON WITH PEACH-BLACKBERRY CHUTNEY

When I think of summer, I think of New England seafood, the smell of the charcoal grill and picnic table dinners with my family when I was growing up. When I'm feeling nostalgic and want a taste of that I make this: easy oven-roasted salmon with a zesty, flavorful chutney. It's impressive enough to serve to guests, but easy enough to toss together as a weeknight dinner. The sweet chutney and spice rub create an energetic flavor dichotomy in this dish that never fails to satisfy.

Serves: 4

FOR THE CHUTNEY

1 tbsp (15 ml) olive oil

4 peaches, peeled and coarsely chopped

2 tbsp (30 ml) red wine vinegar

Pinch of salt

½ cup (74 g) blackberries

1 tbsp (2 g) fresh thyme

FOR THE SALMON

1 wild-caught salmon filet (about 1½ lbs [680 g])

2 tbsp (30 ml) olive oil

1 tbsp (15 g) coconut sugar

1 clove garlic, minced

2 tsp (4 g) paprika

2 tsp (4 g) chili powder

¼ tsp black pepper

½ tsp sea salt

2 scallions, thinly sliced, for garnish

To make the chutney: Place the olive oil, peaches and vinegar in a saucepan over medium heat. Cook, stirring frequently, for 10 to 12 minutes, or until the peaches are syrupy. Remove from the heat and stir in the salt, blackberries and thyme. Set aside.

Preheat the oven to 375°F (190°C). Line a baking sheet with parchment paper.

To make the salmon: Place the salmon skin side down on the baking sheet and drizzle with olive oil.

In a small bowl, stir together the coconut sugar, garlic, paprika, chili powder, pepper and salt. Rub the spice mixture evenly over the salmon.

Bake for 20 to 22 minutes, until the salmon begins to flake.

Top with peach chutney and sliced scallions.

NOTE: A large piece of salmon will require a longer cooking time and perhaps a lower temperature to avoid drying out. If I'm cooking a filet larger than 2 pounds (907 g), I bake it at 350°F (176°C) for 25 to 30 minutes. Individual salmon pieces cook better at 400°F (204°C) for 15 minutes.

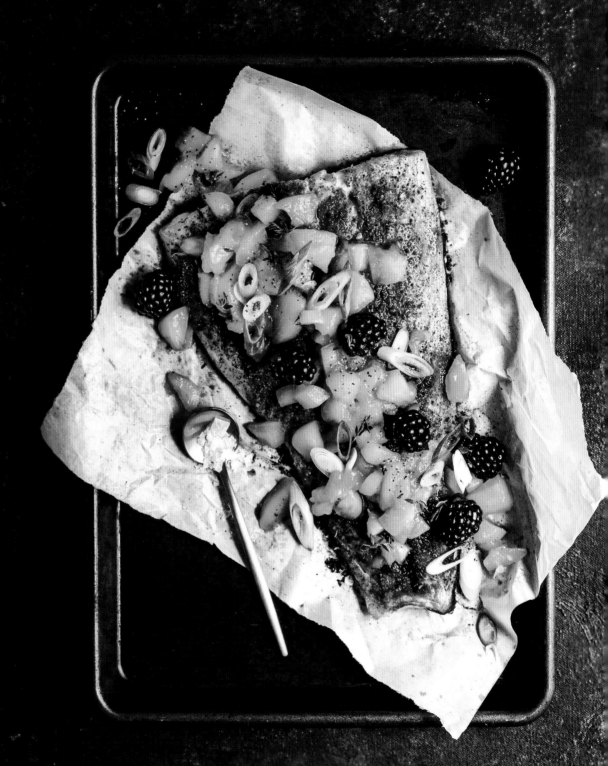

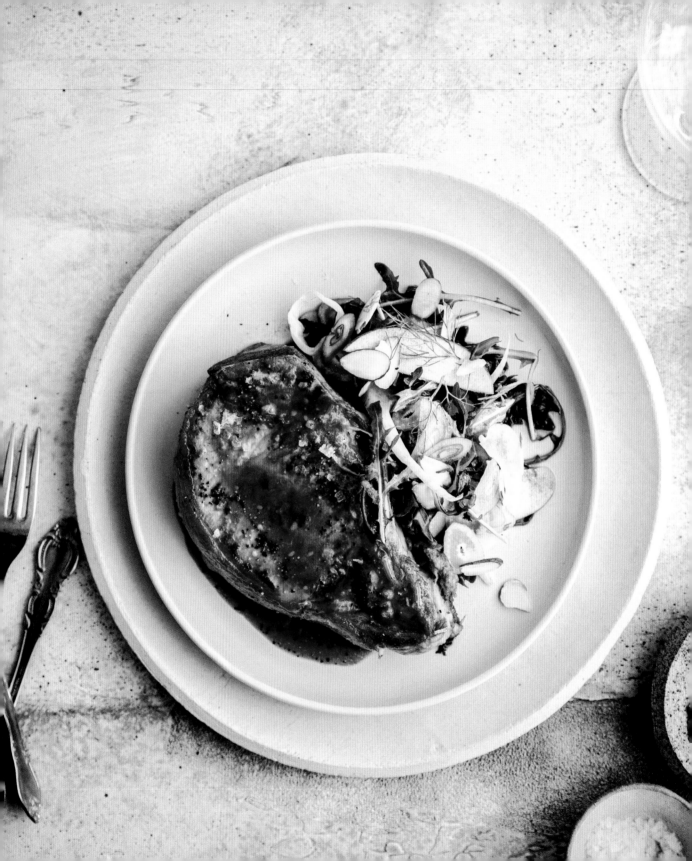

MAPLE-MUSTARD PORK CHOPS WITH APPLE-FENNEL SLAW

This dish is the love child of so many delicious things, but let's start with the pork. I'm sorry to say I wrote off pork until just a couple of years ago, thinking the other white meat was just a bland mistake that my parents used to buy when it was on sale. Since learning how to get a good sear with my favorite Material Kitchen pans, I gave pork chops one last try. I've found that the key is browning them to get a good crispy edge, while making sure they aren't overcooked, then making the sauce with the drippings in the pan while the pork chops rest. I pair them with a tangy apple-fennel slaw. Fennel is a deeply underrated vegetable that is the perfect mild, crunchy pairing with this flavorful pork dish.

Serves: 4

FOR THE SLAW

Juice of ½ lemon

1 tbsp (15 ml) apple cider vinegar

3 tbsp (45 ml) olive oil

¼ tsp sea salt

¼ tsp black pepper

1 shallot, thinly sliced

1 bulb fennel, thinly sliced

1 apple, halved, cored and sliced

1 cup (20 g) arugula

¼ cup (15 g) finely chopped fresh parsley

¼ cup (27 g) sliced almonds

FOR THE PORK CHOPS

4 bone-in pork chops (about 2½ lbs [1.1 kg])

½ tsp sea salt

½ tsp black pepper

2 tbsp (30 ml) olive oil

⅓ cup (80 ml) chicken broth

3 tbsp (45 ml) maple syrup

2 tbsp (30 ml) Dijon mustard

1 tbsp (15 ml) balsamic vinegar

To make the slaw: Whisk together the lemon juice, apple cider vinegar, oil, salt and pepper. Add the shallot to the dressing and set it aside.

Toss together the fennel, apple, arugula and parsley. Pour the shallot dressing over the vegetables and coat evenly. Top with the almonds and set aside.

To make the pork chops: Heat a large skillet over medium-high heat. Season the pork chops with salt and pepper. Add the oil to the skillet, then add the pork chops and cook for 6 to 7 minutes on each side, until a thermometer reads 135°F (57°C). Move the cooked pork chops to a plate and set aside.

Pour the broth into the skillet, then whisk in the maple syrup, mustard and balsamic vinegar. Whisk and simmer for 4 to 5 minutes, until the sauce is thickened. Turn off the heat and immediately add the cooked pork chops to the hot skillet to coat in the sauce.

Plate the pork chops and serve with the apple-fennel slaw and an extra drizzle of the sauce.

NOTE: Depending on the size of your pan you may want to sear your pork chops two at a time to ensure they get a good, crispy sear on the edges.

COCONUT MILK–BRAISED CHICKEN AND SWEET POTATO

Part of the problem with being a food photographer is that by the time dinner rolls around I want nothing to do with cooking. The kitchen is finally clean and I've washed dozens of dishes, and I'm just over it. It's all I can do on a weekly basis to not run out for some bone broth at the shop up the street and call it a night. Quick and easy stovetop meals with minimal ingredients are how I talk myself into cooking dinner, which makes this Coconut Milk–Braised Chicken and Sweet Potato a staple in my life. It's delicious over a bed of cauliflower rice or rice to add something extra to the meal!

Serves: 4

FOR THE CHICKEN AND SWEET POTATO

2 tbsp (30 ml) olive oil

1 lb (454 g) boneless skinless chicken breasts or thighs, diced into 2-inch (5-cm) pieces

1 (1-inch [2.5-cm]) piece fresh ginger, grated

2 cloves garlic, minced

1 large sweet potato, diced

1 zucchini or summer squash, sliced into half moons

1 (14-oz [413-ml]) can full-fat coconut milk

1½ cups (360 ml) chicken broth

2 tbsp (30 ml) coconut aminos

½ tsp chili powder

½ tsp ground turmeric

Juice of 1 lime

¼ cup (15 g) fresh basil

½ tsp red pepper flakes (optional)

FOR SERVING

2 cups (372 g) cooked rice or cauliflower rice

¼ cup (15 g) fresh cilantro

Lime wedges

To make the chicken and sweet potato: Heat the oil in a large pot over medium heat. Add the chicken and sear on each side for 2 to 3 minutes. Add the ginger, garlic and sweet potato. Stir and cook for 4 minutes, then add the zucchini and stir to combine.

Pour in the coconut milk, broth and coconut aminos, then stir in the chili powder, turmeric, lime juice, basil and red pepper flakes (if using). Bring to a simmer, then reduce the heat to low and simmer for about 20 minutes, or until the chicken is cooked through and the potatoes are soft.

To serve: Serve the chicken over rice topped with cilantro and extra lime wedges.

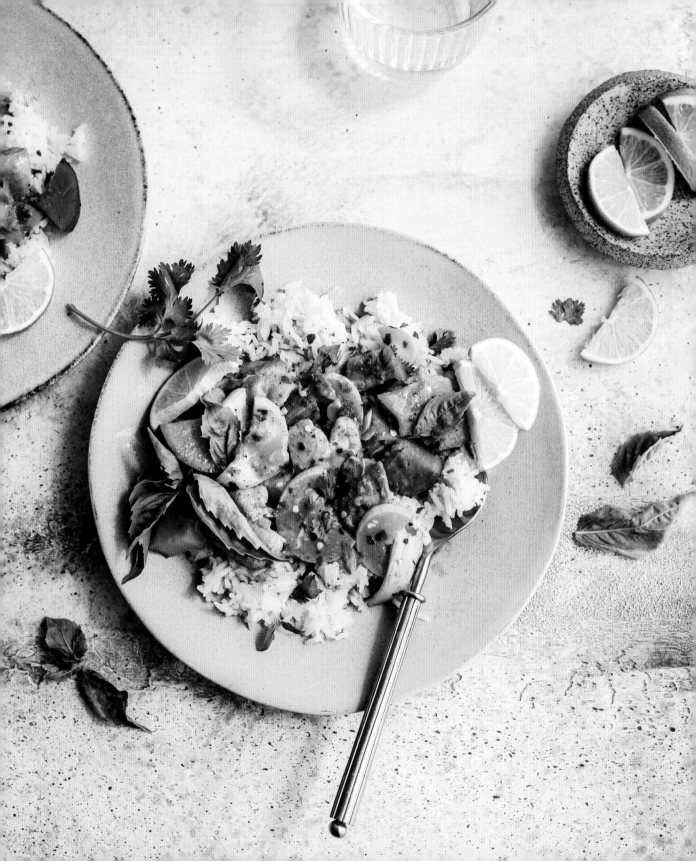

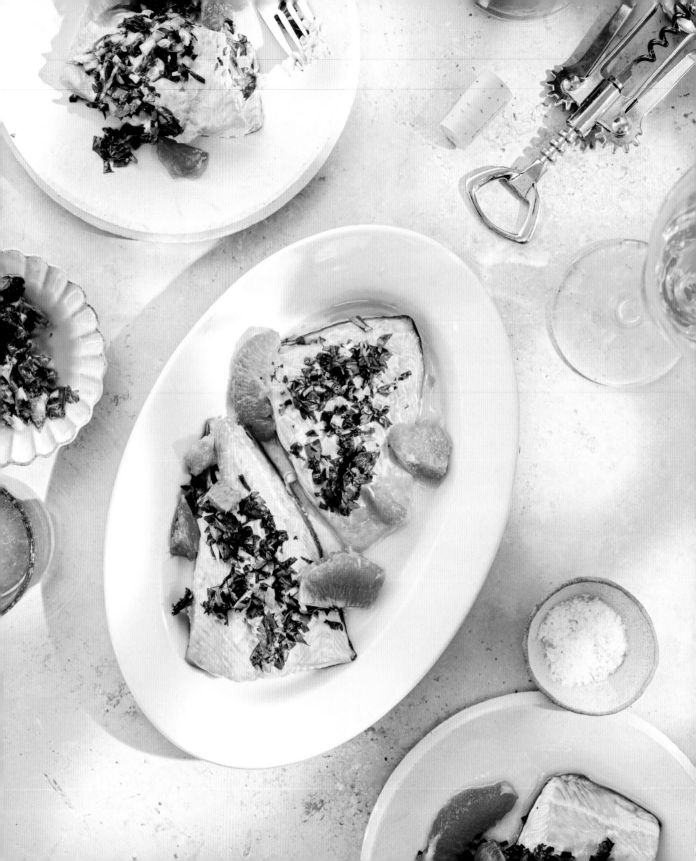

ARCTIC CHAR WITH LEMON SALSA VERDE AND GRAPEFRUIT

My maiden voyage with arctic char took place in a tiny tapas restaurant on the edge of Reykjavík where I'd gone to ring in the New Year with my dad. We mostly ate eggs and steamed vegetables in our Airbnb that trip, but the arctic char I had in that one restaurant stands out like ink on sheets in my mind. I remember little of how it was prepared, only that the fish was so buttery and moist that I knew I needed to learn how to cook it myself back home. Here I've paired it with a citrusy salsa verde and juicy grapefruit. It's light and refreshing while also being perfectly satisfying and fancy enough to serve to guests.

Serves: 4

FOR THE LEMON SALSA VERDE

1 shallot, minced

2 cloves garlic, minced

Juice of ½ lemon

⅓ cup (80 ml) olive oil

¼ tsp sea salt

½ cup (30 g) finely chopped fresh parsley

¼ cup (15 g) finely chopped fresh cilantro

2 tbsp (6 g) chopped fresh chives

FOR THE ARCTIC CHAR

1 lb (454 g) arctic char filets

1 tbsp (15 ml) olive oil

¼ tsp sea salt

FOR SERVING

1 grapefruit, peeled and segmented

To make the lemon salsa verde: Whisk together the shallot, garlic, lemon juice, oil and salt. Stir in the parsley, cilantro and chives. Set aside.

To make the arctic char: Heat the oven on broil and line a baking sheet with parchment paper. Place the fish on the baking sheet, drizzle evenly with oil and sprinkle with salt. Broil for 7 minutes, until the fish is flakey.

To serve: Plate the arctic char and serve it with a spoonful of salsa verde and grapefruit segments.

CHIMICHURRI CHICKEN SKEWERS

One of my proudest accomplishments has been getting my parents hard-core addicted to chimichurri. You've probably had chimichurri served over a steak, but it's also a kismet companion to chicken, fish and any other savory item you want to put on the grill, which makes it perfect for these skewers.

Serves: 4

FOR THE CHIMICHURRI

1 cup (60 g) finely chopped fresh parsley

½ cup (30 g) finely chopped fresh cilantro

⅓ cup (80 ml) olive oil

2 tbsp (30 ml) red wine vinegar

2 cloves garlic, minced

½ tsp sea salt

¼ tsp red pepper flakes (optional)

FOR THE SKEWERS

1 lb (454 g) chicken breast, diced into 1-inch (2.5-cm) cubes

1 cup (150 g) cherry tomatoes

1 zucchini, shaved into ribbons

1 red onion, cut into wedges

1 cup (70 g) baby bella mushrooms

To make the chimichurri: In a medium-sized bowl, stir together the parsley, cilantro, oil, vinegar, garlic, salt and red pepper flakes (if using). Place one-third of the sauce in a gallon zip-top bag and set the rest aside.

To make the skewers: Add the chicken to the bag and toss to coat, then allow it to marinate in the fridge for 1 to 2 hours.

Preheat a grill or a lightly greased grill pan on a stove. Thread the skewers with the chicken and vegetables, alternating ingredients as you go. When threading the zucchini, bunch it up like an accordion and place it on the skewer. The recipe will fill six to eight skewers, depending on the length.

Grill for 5 to 7 minutes on each side, or until the chicken is cooked. Serve topped with the remaining chimichurri.

NOTE: If you don't have access to a grill, bake these in the oven on a sheet pan at 425°F (218°C) for 20 to 25 minutes. If desired, broil for 2 minutes for an extra-crisp finish.

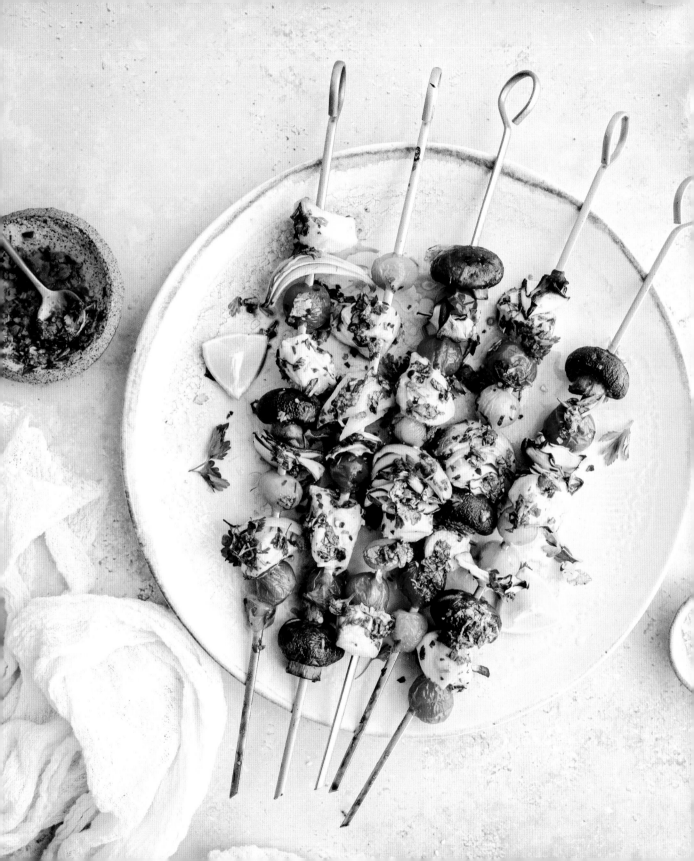

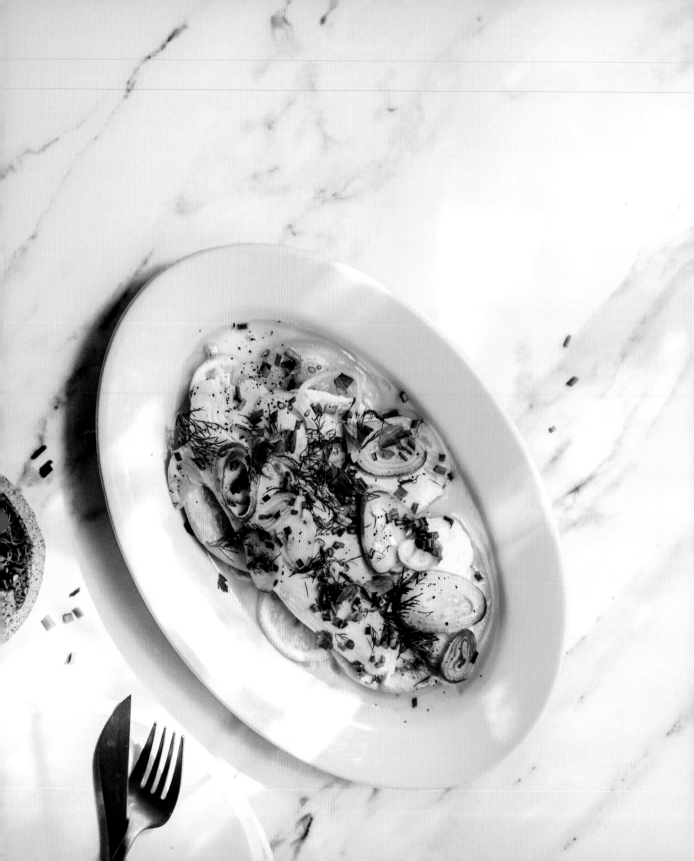

CITRUSY HERB-AND-SHALLOT FISH BAKE

This is not a fish recipe. This is a love letter to citrus and herbs written by the granddaughter of a fisherman. But it's not a Romeo-and-Juliet type of love story. This one has no plot twist, no family drama, no other-shoe-dropping threat. It's all rainbows and maybe the faint sound of Bing Crosby singing in the background. Unrealistic? Maybe, but miracles do happen sometimes.

Serves: 4

2 tbsp (30 ml) olive oil

2 lemons, 1 juiced and 1 thinly sliced

2 oranges,1 juiced and 1 thinly sliced

1 large white fish filet (about 1 lb [454 g])

2 large shallots, thinly sliced

¼ cup (15 g) finely chopped fresh parsley, divided

2 tbsp (6 g) finely chopped fresh chives, divided

2 tbsp (6 g) finely chopped fresh dill, divided

½ tsp sea salt

½ tsp black pepper

Preheat the oven to 425°F (218°C). Lay a large piece of parchment paper on a rimmed baking sheet.

Whisk together the oil, lemon juice and orange juice in a small bowl.

Place the lemon and orange slices on one side of the parchment paper in an even layer about the length of the fish filet. Lay the filet over the citrus slices, then scatter the shallots on and around the fish.

Drizzle the citrus oil over the fish, then top with half of the parsley, chives and dill. Add the salt and pepper. Fold half of the parchment over the fish and tuck the edges of the parchment in tightly to seal.

Place the baking sheet in the oven and bake for 10 to 12 minutes, or until the fish is opaque and flakey. Top with the remaining herbs.

CITRUS ROASTED CHICKEN THIGHS WITH ARTICHOKES

I like chicken thighs on a level that is probably abnormal. Which is to say, I'd eat them plain with some roasted veggies every night without complaint. But I panic when I need to cook chicken for someone else, because most people have higher standards than I do. Luckily, a little citrus and some spices go a long way on planet chicken. Toss in some artichokes and a spoonful of romesco, and you've got a meal that is downright gourmet while hardly even trying.

Serves: 4 to 6

FOR THE CHICKEN

2 tsp (3 g) sumac

Juice of 1 orange

Juice of 1 lemon

2 tbsp (30 ml) olive oil

½ tsp paprika

½ tsp garlic powder

¼ tsp black pepper

½ tsp sea salt

6 bone-in chicken thighs (about 2 lbs [907 g])

1 shallot, thinly sliced

1 (14-oz [400-g]) can artichoke hearts, drained and halved

FOR SERVING

1 batch Nut-Free Romesco (page 129)

Fresh thyme

To make the chicken: Stir together the sumac, orange juice, lemon juice, oil, paprika, garlic powder, pepper and salt in a gallon zip-top bag. Add the chicken to the marinade and place in the fridge for 30 minutes to 2 hours.

Preheat the oven to 425°F (218°C) and lightly grease a large, oven-safe skillet. Pour the chicken and marinade into the prepared skillet and arrange the shallot and artichoke hearts around the chicken.

Place the skillet in the oven and bake for 40 minutes, or until the chicken reaches 165°F (74°C).

To serve: Plate the chicken with artichoke hearts over a scoop of romesco. Garnish with fresh thyme.

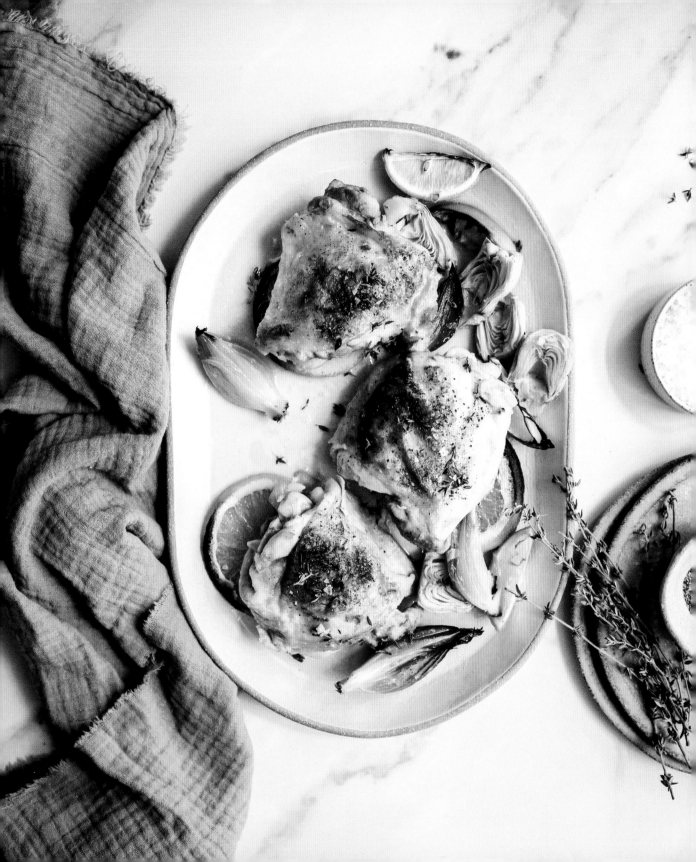

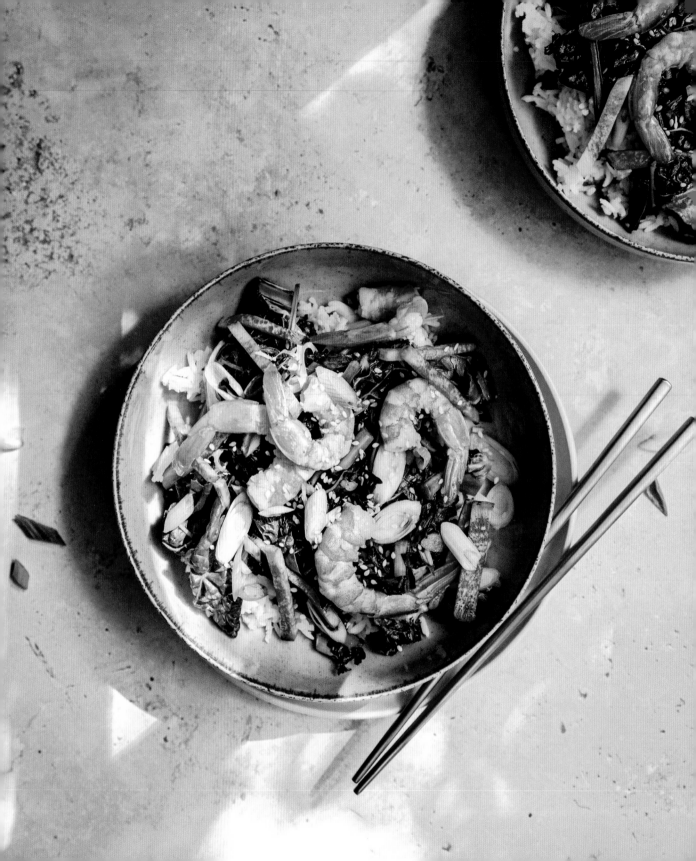

WILTED GREENS AND SHRIMP STIR-FRY

Despite my New England roots, I'm undeniably a New Yorker. I do things fast, I work long hours and I'm pretty impatient. I also have zero counter space and one of those tiny apartment ovens that is only one step above an easy bake oven. All of this is to say, I need meals that can cook fast with minimal cookware and ingredients because there is just no time and no space for anything complicated. In other words, I thrive on stir-fry, and this is one of my favorites.

Serves: 4

FOR THE STIR-FRY

2 tbsp (27 g) coconut oil

2 cloves garlic, minced

1 (2-inch [5-cm]) piece fresh ginger, grated

1 lb (454 g) large shrimp

3 tbsp (45 ml) coconut aminos

1 tbsp (15 ml) rice vinegar

¼ cup (60 ml)) chicken broth

6 cups (402 g) greens of choice, such as kale, spinach, chard, etc.

2 radishes, julienned

¼ cup (15 g) finely chopped fresh cilantro

FOR SERVING

2 cups (372 g) cooked rice or cauliflower rice

4 scallions, thinly sliced

1 tbsp (9 g) sesame seeds

To make the stir-fry: Place the oil in a large skillet over medium-high heat. Add the garlic and ginger, and sauté for 2 minutes. Add the shrimp in an even layer and sear for 2 minutes on each side, until opaque. Pour in the coconut aminos, vinegar and broth. Sauté for 2 to 3 minutes, then remove the shrimp to a plate.

Add the greens to the skillet and sauté in the remaining sauce for 5 to 7 minutes, or until wilted. Add the shrimp back to the skillet and mix with the greens, then remove from the heat and stir in the radishes and cilantro.

To serve: Divide the stir-fry into four bowls with rice. Top with scallions and sesame seeds.

BRAISED BEEF RAGU

New York restaurants taught me that ragu is not just a brand of sauce: ragu is a way of life. It's also an easy-yet-gourmet dinner situation that warms you down to your bones. You can make it in an oven or a slow cooker. Serve it over anything from pasta or polenta to mashed potatoes, and it's a winner every time.

Serves: 6

2 tbsp (30 ml) olive oil

2 lbs (907 g) beef chuck roast, cut into 4–5 pieces

½ tsp sea salt

¼ tsp black pepper

2 large shallots, sliced

4 cloves garlic, minced

2 large carrots, peeled and roughly chopped

1 rib celery, chopped

¼ cup (60 ml) balsamic vinegar

1 cup (240 ml) red wine

1 cup (240 ml) beef bone broth

1 (28-oz [793-g]) can San Marzano tomatoes with liquid

2 tbsp (2 g) fresh thyme, plus more for garnish

FOR SERVING

½ lb (227 g) pasta, cooked according to package directions

Fresh mozzarella or grated Parmesan (optional)

If you are using an oven, preheat it to 325°F (163°C).

Place the oil in a large Dutch oven over medium-high heat. Sprinkle the beef with the salt and pepper. Add it to the pot and brown for 3 minutes on each side. Remove the browned beef to a plate and set it aside.

Add the shallots and garlic to the pot, and sauté for 2 minutes. Add the carrots and celery, and sauté for 4 to 5 minutes, until tender. Pour in the vinegar and red wine, using it to deglaze the bottom of the pot.

If you are using an oven, add the broth, tomatoes and thyme, then return the beef to the pot. Place the pot in the oven and cook for 2½ hours. Once cooked, remove the beef from the pot and shred it, then stir it back into the sauce.

If you are using a slow cooker, after deglazing, scrape the contents of the pot into a slow cooker. Add the broth, tomatoes and thyme, then add the browned beef to the slow cooker. Cover and cook on low for 6 to 8 hours. Once cooked, remove the beef from the pot and shred it, then stir it back into the sauce.

To serve: Serve the ragu over the cooked pasta garnished with extra thyme and fresh mozzarella, if desired.

NOTE: Depending on the cooking method you choose, your ragu might be more liquidy. If you prefer a thicker ragu, simmer it uncovered on the stovetop until the liquid is reduced—about 10 minutes does the trick.

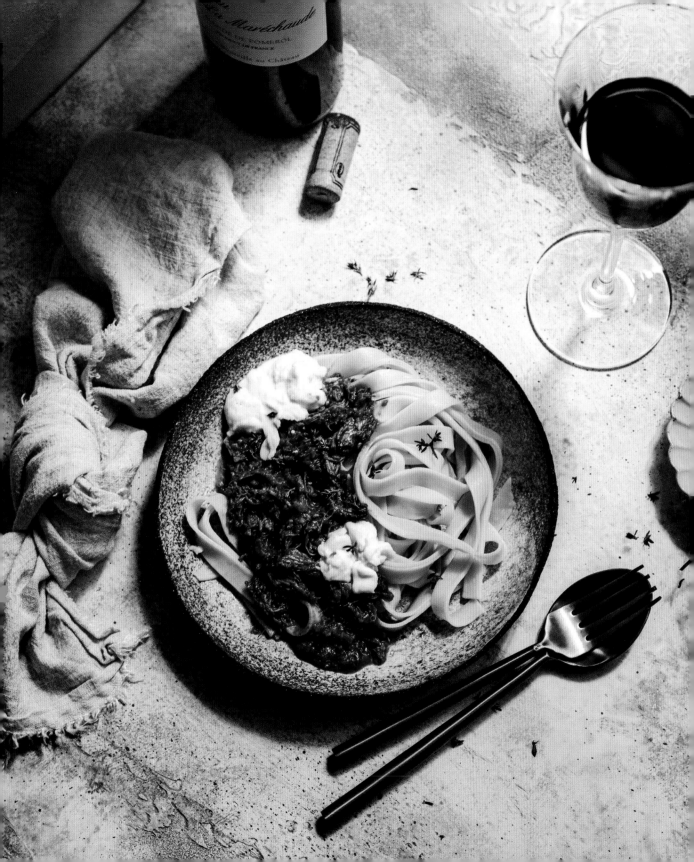

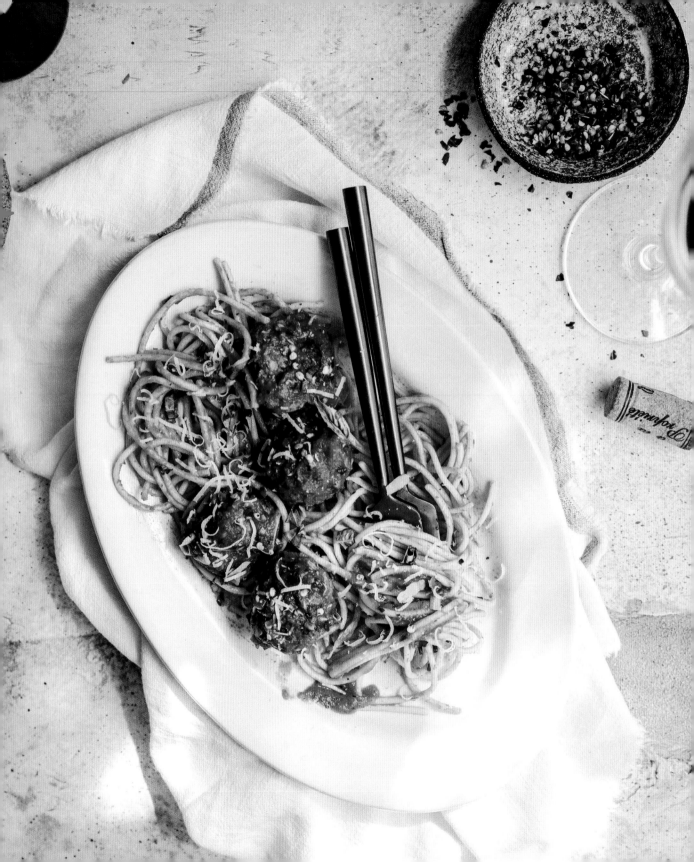

HARISSA MEATBALLS

You know what gets really exciting when you're an adult? Leftovers. Sweet, sweet leftovers. They're one of my favorite things, along with early bird dinners and grocery store sales. And meatballs? Well, meatballs are the best leftover food. Pop them in a saucepan and heat them up and they're just as good, if not better, than they were the first day. This recipe purposely calls for more ingredients than my other recipes, so you're bound to have leftovers on hand for a few days. You can thank me later when your meatballs are reheating. Please note that you'll want to make my Apartment Arrabbiata (page 125) in advance; this will help the harissa sauce come together in no time at all.

Serves: 8

FOR THE MEATBALLS

1 lb (454 g) ground beef

1 lb (454 g) ground turkey

¼ cup (40 g) finely chopped onion

4 cloves garlic, minced

½ tsp sea salt

1 tsp paprika

2 tbsp (8 g) finely chopped fresh parsley

1 egg

1 tbsp (8 g) cassava flour

FOR THE HARISSA SAUCE

2–4 tbsp (32–64 g) harissa paste

2 tsp (4 g) paprika

1 batch of Apartment Arrabbiata (page 125)

½ cup (120 ml) water

Preheat the oven to 400°F (204°C).

To make the meatballs: Stir together the beef, turkey, onion, garlic, salt, paprika, parsley, egg and flour in a large bowl until well combined. Pro tip: Use your hands for this one!

Roll the mixture into about 16 to 20 meatballs and place them 1 inch (2.5 cm) apart on a baking sheet. Bake for 12 minutes.

While the meatballs are baking, make the harissa sauce: Stir together the harissa, paprika, arrabbiata and water in a large pot. Bring the sauce to a boil, then reduce to a simmer.

Place the cooked meatballs in the harissa sauce and simmer for at least 30 minutes, then enjoy!

NOTE: Store these meatballs in the fridge for up to 5 days, or freeze in an airtight container. Thaw and reheat them in a saucepan when desired.

TOMATO-OLIVE BAKED CHICKEN

One of the great struggles of "adulting" is figuring out what to cook on a weeknight. It's a laborious task that we all face on a pretty regular basis and, as much as I like creative cooking, I hate weeknight chicken puzzles as much as the next busy individual. The game changer? Figuring out one-pan dishes with some well-chosen herbs and vegetables that turn monotonous chicken into a delicious, satisfying meal. Pop that pan in the oven and you've got your whole meal ready to go, along with a few days of leftovers if you fly solo like me.

Serves: 4 to 6

2 tbsp (30 ml) olive oil

6 boneless chicken thighs (about 1½ lbs [680 g])

½ tsp sea salt

½ tsp black pepper

2 shallots, sliced in half

2 cloves garlic, minced

½ cup (120 ml) dry white wine

2 cups (300 g) cherry tomatoes, halved

½ cup (90 g) Greek olives, pitted

2 tbsp (2 g) fresh thyme

1 lemon, thinly sliced

½ cup (30 g) chopped fresh basil

Preheat the oven to 425°F (218°C).

Add the oil to a large skillet over medium-high heat. Season the chicken thighs with salt and pepper. Add them to the skillet and sear for 2 to 3 minutes on each side. Remove to a plate and set aside. Keep them skin side up, if using skin.

Add the shallots and garlic to the pan, and sauté for 1 minute. Pour in the white wine and simmer, stirring, for 2 minutes.

Return the chicken to the skillet along with the tomatoes, olives and thyme. Nestle lemon slices around the chicken, then place in the oven and bake for 15 minutes, or until the chicken is cooked through. Top with fresh basil to serve.

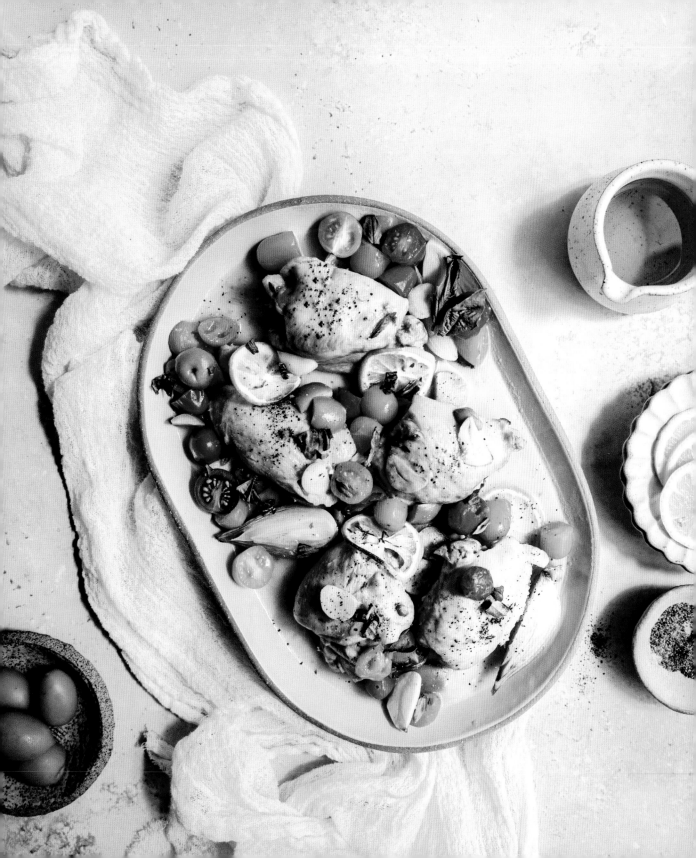

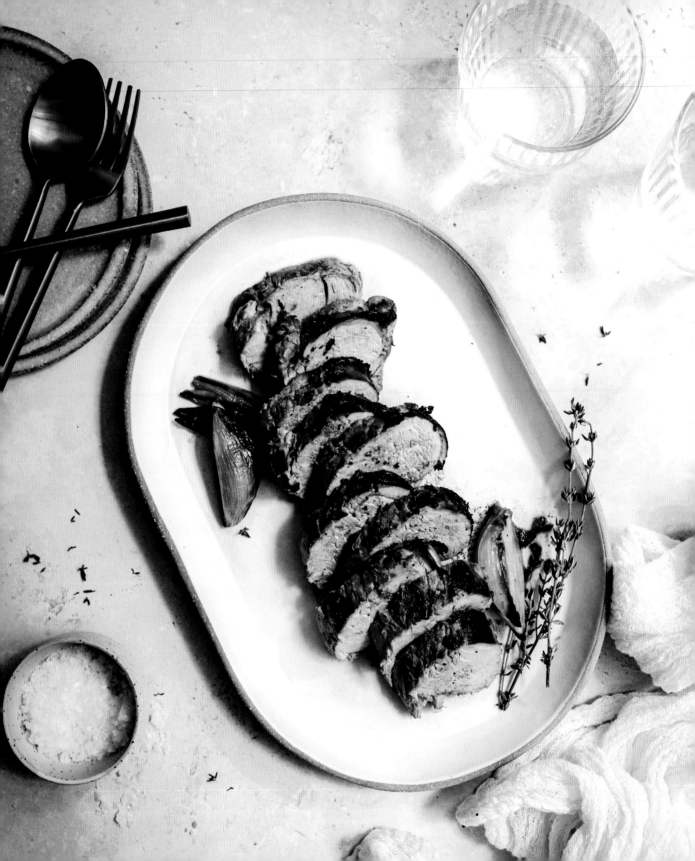

CITRUS PORK TENDERLOIN

My family refers to really good food as "extravagant gifts of deliciousness," and it's not a term that is awarded to very many things. This pork though? This pork gets the title. It's best to marinate overnight so the citrusy magic has plenty of time to do its work. In terms of serving, you don't need much other than some roasted vegetables because the pork is already so flavorful and addictive. This is also the perfect dish to make for company since you can easily double the recipe and it cooks up in less than twenty minutes.

Serves: 4

2 shallots, sliced in quarters

2 cloves garlic, minced

Juice of 1 orange

Juice and zest of 1 lemon

2 tbsp (30 ml) olive oil

½ tsp sea salt

½ tsp black pepper

2 tbsp (30 ml) balsamic vinegar

1 large or 2 small pork tenderloin (totaling about 1½ lbs [681 g])

Fresh thyme, for garnish

Mix the shallots, garlic, orange juice, lemon juice and zest, oil, salt, pepper and vinegar in a gallon zip-top bag. Add the pork tenderloin to the bag and place it in the fridge to marinate for at least 2 hours or overnight.

Heat the oven on broil and place the pork on a baking sheet along with the shallots. Cook about 4 inches (10 cm) below the broiler for 12 to 15 minutes, or until the pork's internal temperature reaches 145°F (63°C). Cover the pork with tinfoil and set aside to rest for 5 minutes before slicing.

Serve the pork thinly sliced with a garnish of fresh thyme and juices from the pan. Plate with the roasted shallots for an extra visual garnish.

FISH PUTTANESCA

I grew up reading *A Series of Unfortunate Events* repeatedly, and Lemony Snicket made me want to be an author. If you've ever read the series, you know that puttanesca is a key part of the first book. But the only unfortunate thing about puttanesca is the number of years it took me to actually make it. Now everything is finally coming full circle. I'm an author, and I've finally made puttanesca a staple in my food life: seafood edition. I use a half-batch of my go-to Apartment Arrabbiata (page 125) for the sauce, and add whatever white fish is readily available. The result is an easy-yet-impressive weeknight meal that also becomes excellent leftovers.

Serves: 4

½ batch Apartment Arrabbiata (page 125)

½ cup (90 g) olives, pitted (I use a mix of green and Castelvetrano.)

2 tbsp (15 g) capers

1 cup (60 g) chopped fresh basil, divided

1 lb (454 g) cod or halibut filets

1 cup (150 g) cherry tomatoes

½ tsp black pepper

Pinch of red pepper flakes

Preheat the oven to 400°F (204°C).

Bring the arrabbiata to a simmer in a large, oven-safe skillet over medium heat. Stir in the olives, capers and half of the basil, then add the fish filets to the top of the sauce.

Sprinkle the tomatoes, pepper and red pepper flakes on top of the fish. Place the skillet in the oven. Bake for 7 to 10 minutes, or until the fish is flakey.

Serve topped with the remaining basil.

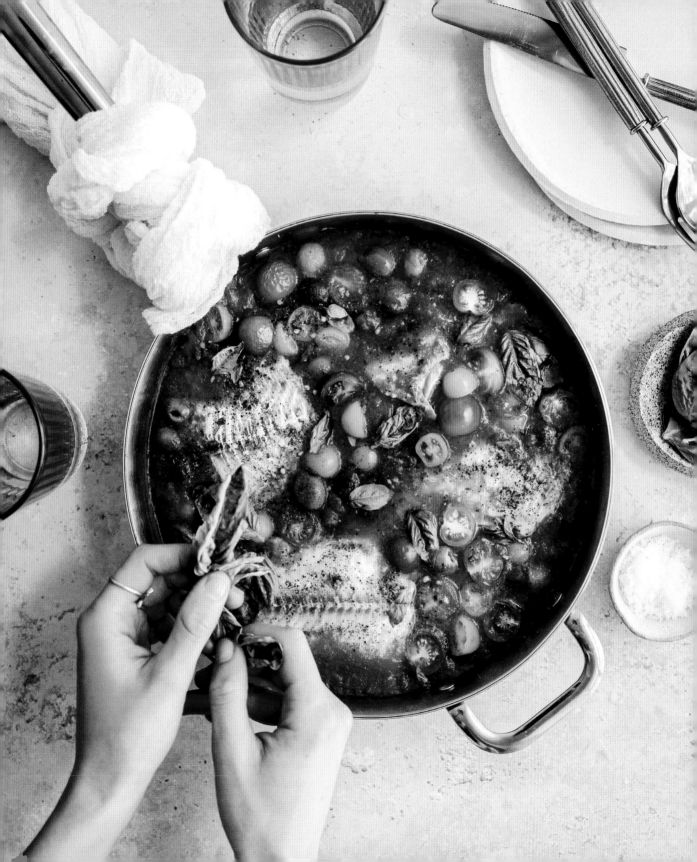

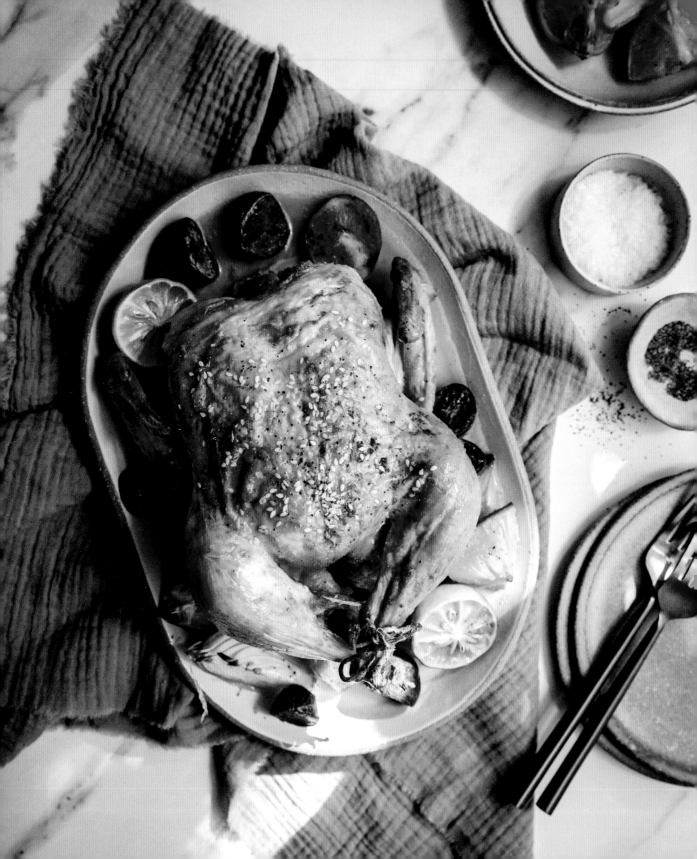

GINGER ROASTED WHOLE CHICKEN AND ROOTS

Cutting into a whole roasted chicken feels like an event, and I'm all about deceptively easy meals that make weeknights feel more special. The extra good news is this recipe also yields excellent leftovers. Here I've roasted the chicken with a bounty of my favorite root vegetables, though you can use whatever roots you prefer and you'll still have a successful one-pan meal ready to go.

Serves: 6

1 (4–5 lbs [1.8–2.2 kg]) whole chicken

4 tbsp (60 ml) olive oil, divided

1 (2-inch [5-cm]) piece fresh ginger, peeled and grated

2 cloves garlic, minced

2 tbsp (30 ml) coconut aminos

1 tsp sea salt, divided

½ tsp black pepper

1 tbsp (8 g) sesame seeds

1 orange, quartered

1 large purple sweet potato, diced into 1-inch (2.5-cm) cubes

1 large Yukon gold potato, diced into 1-inch (2.5-cm) cubes

1 lb (454 g) carrots, peeled and roughly chopped

1 onion, quartered

1 large parsnip, peeled and chopped

Preheat the oven to 425°F (218°C). Place the chicken in a rimmed baking dish.

In a medium-sized bowl, stir together 2 tablespoons (30 ml) of the oil, the ginger, garlic, coconut aminos, ½ teaspoon of salt and the pepper.

Rub the ginger mixture all over the chicken and underneath the skin. Sprinkle the sesame seeds over the top of the chicken. Place the orange in the cavity, then tie the legs together.

Toss the potatoes, carrots, onion and parsnip in the bowl with the remaining oil and salt. Scatter the vegetables around the chicken in the pan.

Place the pan in the oven and roast for 15 minutes. Reduce the heat to 350°F (177°C) and roast for 1 hour, or for 15 minutes per pound (454 g).

Allow the chicken to rest for 10 to 20 minutes, tented with tinfoil, then slice and enjoy!

NOTE: To make this strict-Paleo, use two sweet potatoes and omit the gold potato.

CITRUS-HERB ROASTED SALMON WITH GARDEN PESTO

This may be my favorite way to cook fish: roasted with citrus and topped with an herbaceous garden pesto. I could eat it again, and again and the fresh, flavorful toppings would rope me in every time. This recipe is yours to own; use whatever pesto recipe and bounty of fresh garden vegetables you'd like to top it off. Just one tip: go double or nothing on the pesto. There's never a case where you can possibly use too much.

Serves: 4

FOR THE SALMON

1 wild-caught salmon filet (about 1½ lbs [680 g])

1 tbsp (30 ml) olive oil

Juice of 1 lemon

1 tbsp (30 ml) honey

2 tbsp (8 g) finely chopped fresh parsley

2 tbsp (6 g) chopped fresh chives

½ tsp sea salt

FOR SERVING

1 batch pesto of choice (page 130)

4 small radishes, thinly sliced

½ cup (75 g) sliced cherry tomatoes

¼ cup (15 g) finely chopped fresh parsley or cilantro

Preheat the oven to 375°F (190°C). Line a baking sheet with parchment paper.

To make the salmon: Place the fish filet skin side down on the baking sheet.

In a small bowl, stir together the oil, lemon juice, honey, parsley, chives and salt. Spread the herb mixture evenly over the fish.

Bake for 20 minutes, or until the fish is opaque and begins to flake.

To serve: Spread pesto over the top of the roasted fish and top with radishes, tomatoes and parsley.

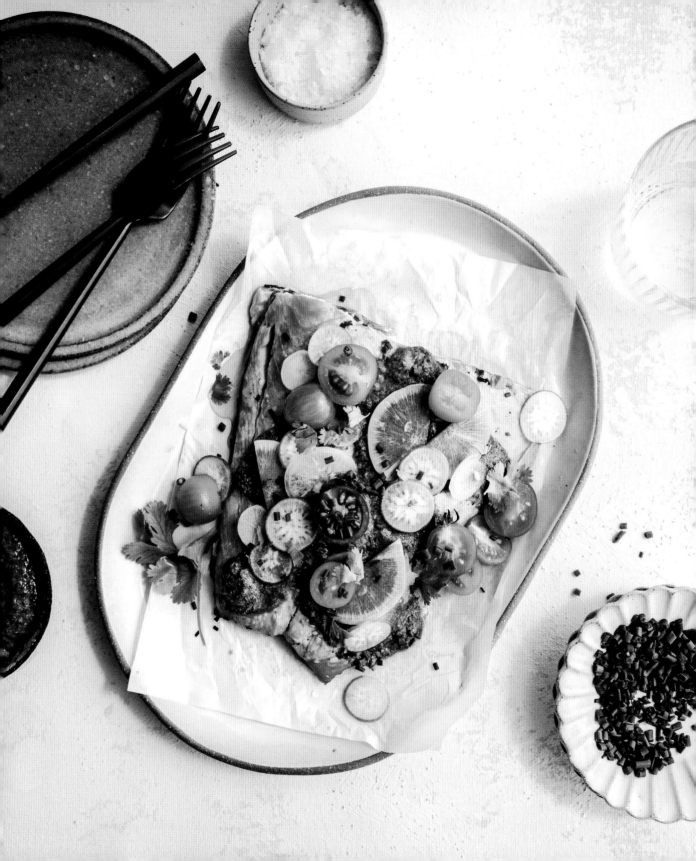

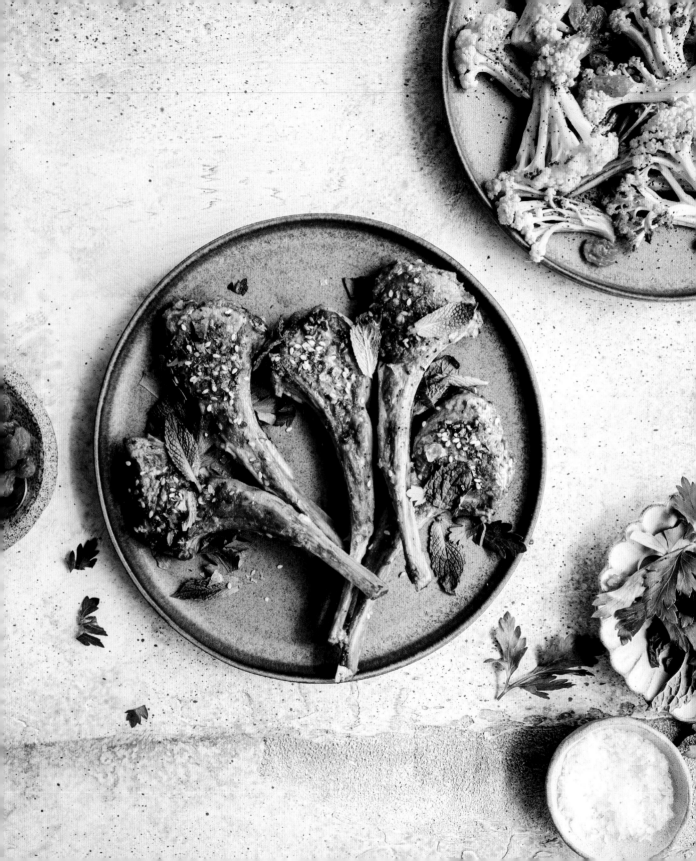

ZA'ATAR LAMB CHOPS WITH CAULIFLOWER AND GOLDEN RAISINS

The first time I ever ate a lamb chop was 2 a.m. on a Monday night—or I guess Tuesday morning! I had just finished the most stressful waitressing shift of my life, and the chef from the restaurant next to mine brought them to me in a to-go container since I was still rolling silverware in the restaurant that had closed four hours ago—it's a long, understaffed story. When I finally got home, I sank to the floor of the kitchen, picked up a lamb chop and swooned. Maybe I was delirious, but I remember thinking it was the best thing I'd ever eaten. Turns out, they're even better when you eat them hot with a delicious sweet-and-salty side dish at a more reasonable dinner hour.

Serves: 4

FOR THE CAULIFLOWER

2 cups (200 g) baby cauliflower florets

2 tbsp (30 ml) olive oil

1 tbsp (15 ml) fresh lemon juice

2 cloves garlic, minced

½ tsp sea salt

¼ cup (36 g) golden raisins

FOR THE ZA'ATAR

2 tbsp (18 g) sesame seeds

2 tbsp (5 g) dried thyme

2 tsp (3 g) ground sumac

1 tsp ground cumin

½ tsp sea salt

FOR THE LAMB

8 lamb chops (about 1½ lbs [680 g])

2 tbsp (30 ml) olive oil

FOR SERVING

Fresh cilantro and mint

Preheat the oven to 400°F (204°C). Line a baking sheet with parchment paper.

To make the cauliflower: Toss the cauliflower florets on the baking sheet with the oil, lemon juice, garlic and salt. Bake for 25 minutes, tossing halfway through. The cauliflower will be golden and crispy. Toss the roasted cauliflower with the golden raisins. Set aside.

To make the za'atar: In a small bowl, stir together the sesame seeds, thyme, sumac, cumin and salt.

To make the lamb: Season the lamb well with the za'atar on each side. Place the oil in a large skillet over medium-high heat. Sear the lamb chops for 2 to 3 minutes on each side, or until you reach the desired level of cooking. Remove the lamb chops from the pan and allow them to rest for 5 minutes.

To serve: Plate the lamb chops alongside the cauliflower and top with fresh herbs.

NOTE: Regular cauliflower works, too, if you don't have baby cauliflower on hand.

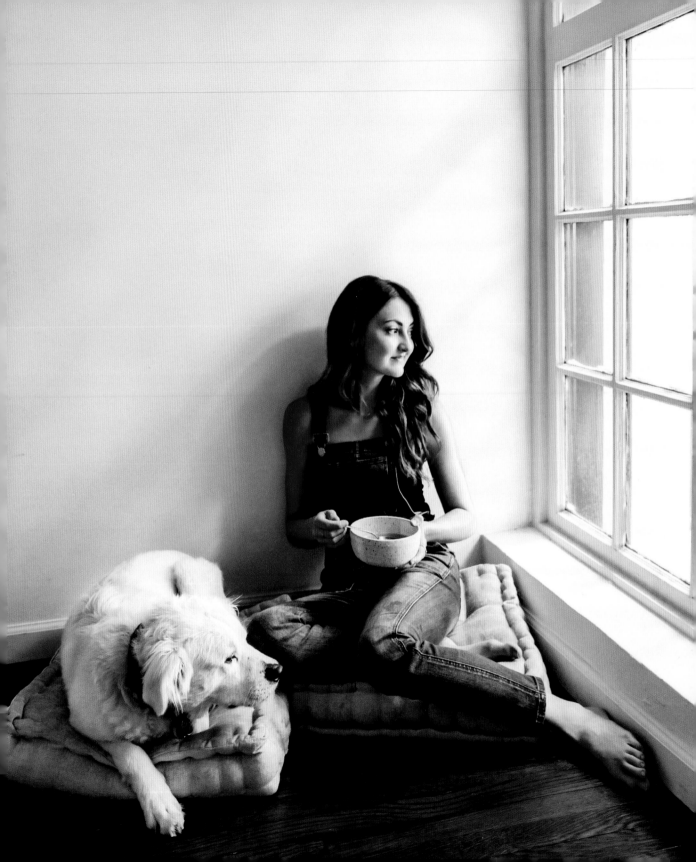

NOURISHING SOUPS AND STEWS

There is a certain feeling in the time between the last days of summer and the first frost of winter, when the ripe fruit falls and the world slips back into the routine of school days and transient weekends. Maybe this is my New England upbringing, but there is a feeling in those weeks that I am forever homesick for, a warmth and familiarity in the changing leaves that always seemed to echo through the rest of the world during autumn. All I want on those days, and whenever I'm dreaming of them, is a large mug of my Spicy Kabocha Soup with Toasted Almonds and Dill (page 57), or my go-to Weeknight Meatball Soup (page 70). This chapter is my best attempt at doing justice to that golden feeling.

BUTTERNUT BEEF STEW

My dream fall day starts with a long walk along the High Line in New York and ends running up the steps of my walk-up to a steaming hot bowl of Butternut Beef Stew and a few reruns of *The Office*. This recipe is one I've perfected over the years in search of a Paleo-friendly stew recipe that didn't lack flavor or texture. My answer was found in the magic combination of braised beef, red wine and tender butternut squash, a.k.a. the flavor combo you never knew you needed.

Serves: 4

FOR THE STEW

2 tbsp (30 ml) olive oil

4 cloves garlic, minced

1½ lbs (680 g) beef stew meat

½ tsp sea salt

½ tsp black pepper

½ sweet onion, diced

1 large parsnip, peeled and roughly sliced

1 tbsp (1 g) fresh thyme, plus more for garnish

1 cup (240 ml) red wine

1 tbsp (16 g) tomato paste

1 quart (960 ml) beef bone broth

2 cups (140 g) sliced baby bella mushrooms

1 medium butternut squash, peeled and cut into 1-inch (2.5-cm) pieces

FOR SERVING

Crusty grain-free bread (optional; I like Against The Grain Baguettes.)

Preheat the oven to 325°F (163°C).

To make the stew: Place the oil in a large Dutch oven over medium-high heat. Add the garlic to the pot, and sauté for 2 minutes. Sprinkle the beef with the salt and pepper. Add it to the pot and brown for 3 minutes on each side. Remove the browned beef to a plate and set it aside.

Add the onion and parsnip to the pot. Sauté, stirring frequently, for 6 to 7 minutes, until the vegetables are tender. Stir in the thyme, red wine, tomato paste and broth. Return the browned beef to the Dutch oven, cover and place in the oven for 1½ hours.

Remove the pot and add the mushrooms and butternut squash. Cover and return the pot to the oven for 1 hour.

To serve: Serve the stew warm garnished with extra thyme and a side of crunchy bread, if desired.

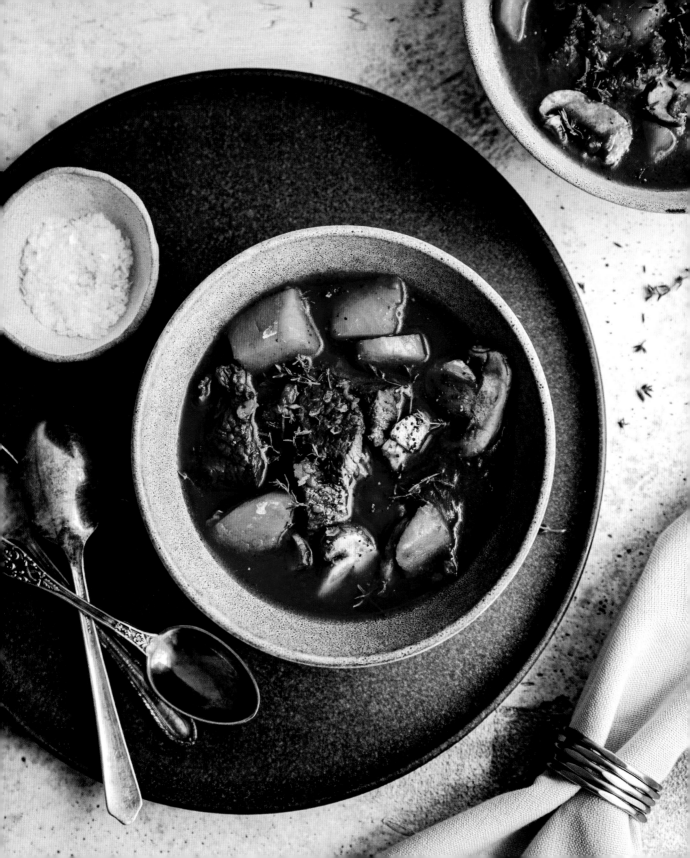

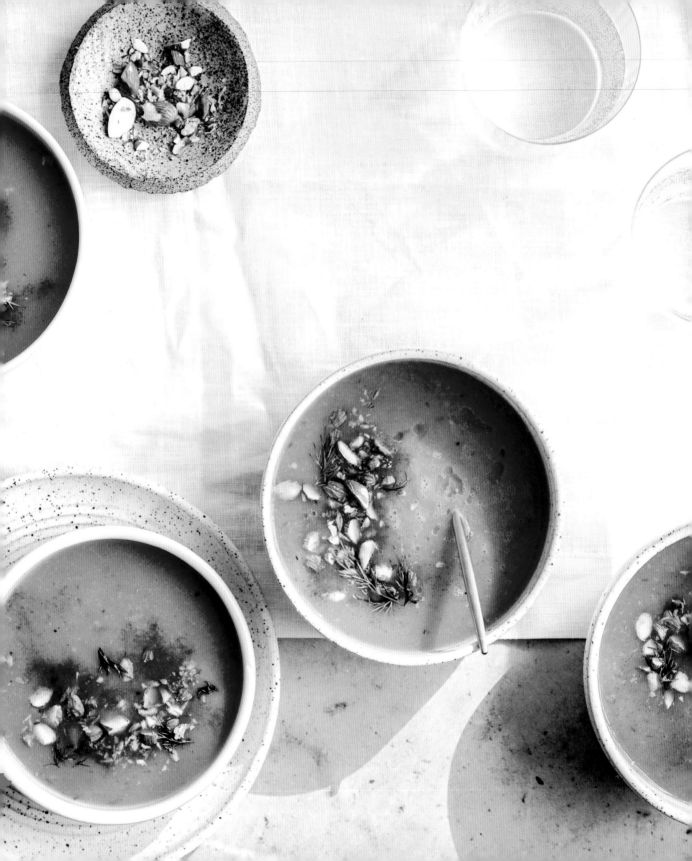

SPICY KABOCHA SOUP WITH TOASTED ALMONDS AND DILL

Squash-based soups may be my ultimate favorite when it comes to the soup world. They're incredibly rich and flavorful despite being the most low-maintenance soup to make, and you can get a bold flavor using only five to ten ingredients you most likely have on hand.

I used my favorite kabocha squash for this soup, but you can easily use butternut or pumpkin depending on what is available to you. I've also used harissa—a Tunisian hot chili pepper paste—to add a spicy kick to this soup. I first encountered harissa in Trader Joe's about four years ago, and it's been a fridge staple ever since. It's the perfect balance of smoky spice with a subtle sweetness that adds depth of flavor without lighting your taste buds ablaze.

Serves: 4

1 large kabocha squash, cut in half with seeds discarded

1 small yellow onion, cut into wedges

1 tbsp (15 ml) melted coconut oil

¼ tsp sea salt

¼ tsp black pepper

½ cup (72 g) chopped almonds

1–2 tbsp (16–32 g) harissa paste, or more for a spicier soup

1 tsp paprika

½ tsp garlic powder

1 quart (960 ml) chicken bone broth

2 tbsp (2 g) chopped fresh dill, for garnish

Preheat the oven to 425°F (218°C). Line a baking sheet with parchment paper.

Drizzle the squash and onion with the coconut oil, then sprinkle with salt and pepper. Place the squash cut side down on the baking sheet along with the onion. Bake for 45 minutes, or until soft.

To toast the almonds, place them in a dry skillet over medium heat. Toast for 4 to 5 minutes, or until golden. Watch carefully to prevent the almonds from burning. Set aside.

Scoop the flesh out of the squash and place it in a blender with the onion, harissa, paprika, garlic powder and broth. Blend until smooth and creamy.

Pour the soup into a large pot and bring to a boil, then reduce to a simmer for 15 minutes to thicken.

Serve topped with the toasted almonds and fresh dill.

NOTE: If you're wary about spice, add just a small spoonful of the harissa paste to start and then add more to taste.

THAI BASIL CHICKEN CURRY

My love affair with Thai curry began years ago with a take-out order while visiting my parents in Connecticut, but blossomed into a fully committed relationship in the tiny, crowded Top Thai Greenwich in New York City. I once ate there seven nights in a row to see if the wonder of the green curry would ever fade in my eyes, but many, many orders and a few years later it still has not. I can never come close to replicating the authentic magic created in that hole-in-the-wall restaurant, but this is the recipe I turn to when the curry craving hits and I've already darkened the door of Top Thai a few too many times that month.

Serves: 4

FOR THE CURRY

1 tbsp (15 ml) coconut oil

1 (1-inch [2.5-cm]) piece fresh ginger, grated

2 cloves garlic, minced

1 lb (454 g) boneless skinless chicken breasts, thinly sliced into strips

1 (13.5-oz [398-ml]) can full-fat coconut milk

1 cup (240 ml) low-sodium chicken broth

3–4 tbsp (45–60 g) red curry paste

½ tsp red pepper flakes (optional)

3 tbsp (45 ml) coconut aminos

2 zucchini, sliced into ribbons or spiralized

1 red bell pepper, thinly sliced

¼ cup (15 g) chopped fresh basil, divided

FOR SERVING

2 cups (372 g) cooked cauliflower rice or jasmine rice

Lime wedges

Sesame seeds

To make the curry: Heat the oil in a large skillet over medium heat. Add the ginger and garlic to the pan. Sauté for 2 to 3 minutes, until fragrant. Add the chicken strips to the skillet and sauté for 6 to 7 minutes, or until no longer pink.

Add the coconut milk, broth, curry paste, red pepper flakes (if using) and coconut aminos. Stir well to combine. Bring the curry to a boil, then reduce to a simmer for 5 minutes. Add the zucchini and bell pepper to the pot. Simmer for 2 to 3 minutes to soften.

To serve: Stir in half of the basil, then divide the curry into four bowls with rice. Top with the remaining basil, lime wedges and sesame seeds.

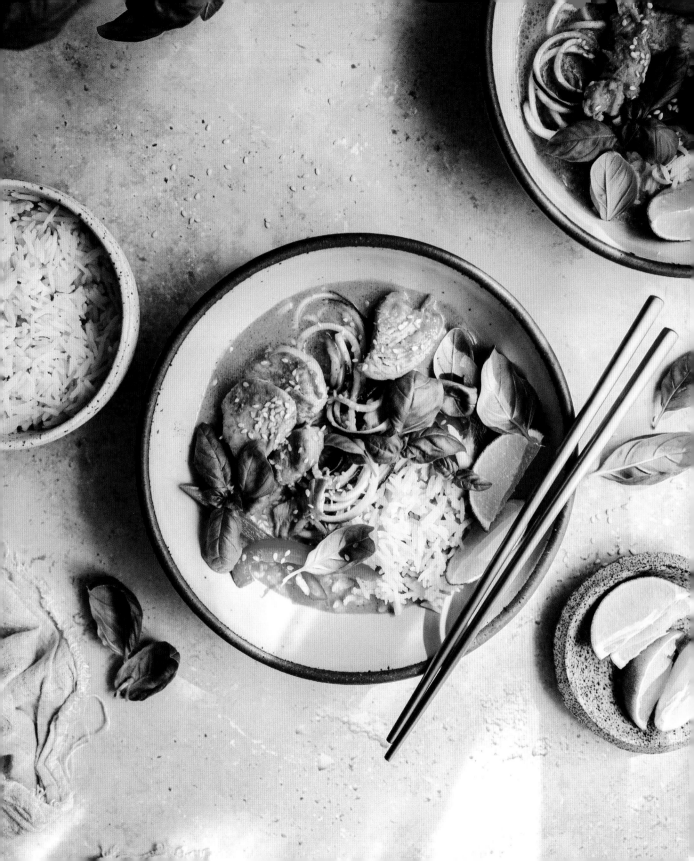

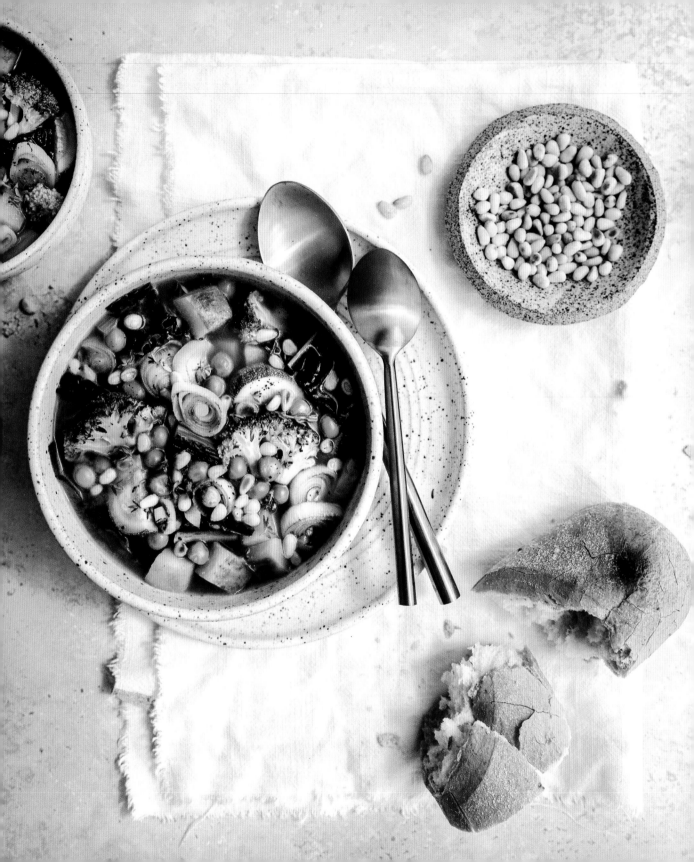

SUMMER GREEN MINESTRONE

My cooking is so largely influenced by New England that it seemed appropriate to make a summer soup. Summer warmth is so transient in that region that a soup is never too far out of the question, especially when the garden greens are overflowing. Minestrone is often seen with pasta or rice, but this Italian soup is really a vehicle for the vegetables that you have on hand. I chose a Paleo version made with summer greens, but this is a great soup to make your own depending on the broths or vegetables you have available.

Serves: 4

2 tbsp (30 ml) extra virgin olive oil

2 cloves garlic, minced

2 shallots, thinly sliced

1 large leek, thinly sliced

2 small zucchini, sliced into half moons

1 large russet potato or white sweet potato, peeled and diced into 1-inch (2.5-cm) pieces

1 quart (960 ml) chicken bone broth

½ cup (46 g) broccoli florets

1 cup (145 g) English peas

2 cups (134 g) kale, roughly chopped

Juice of 1 lemon

½ tsp sea salt

½ tsp black pepper

¼ cup (35 g) pine nuts, toasted (optional)

Heat the oil in a large pot over medium heat. Add the garlic and shallots. Sauté for 2 to 3 minutes, until fragrant. Add the leek, zucchini and potato. Sauté for 6 to 7 minutes, or until softened.

Add the broth, broccoli and peas. Bring the soup to a boil, then reduce the heat and simmer for 10 minutes, until all the vegetables are soft.

Stir in the kale, lemon juice, salt and pepper. Simmer for 3 to 4 minutes to wilt the kale. Divide the soup among four bowls and serve topped with pine nuts (if using).

LEMONGRASS SHRIMP CURRY

Curry is such an easy sell for me no matter what time of year it is or what I have on hand for vegetables and protein. I'm often at the mercy of a jar of curry paste for flavoring my curry, so I like to make this homemade lemongrass paste to change things up when I have a little extra time. It makes it taste just a little bit more like the elusive Thai restaurant curry.

Serves: 4

FOR THE LEMONGRASS CURRY PASTE

2 stalks lemongrass, chopped with tough outer layers removed

1 shallot, chopped

1 serrano chili, sliced and destemmed

1 (1-inch [2.5-cm]) piece fresh ginger, peeled and chopped

2 cloves garlic

¼ cup (15 g) fresh basil

2 tbsp (30 ml) olive oil

1 tbsp (15 ml) lime juice

½ tsp sea salt

½ tsp black pepper

FOR THE CURRY

1 tbsp (15 ml) olive oil

1 lb (454 g) large shrimp

1 cup (110 g) thin green beans

1 (13.5-oz [398-ml]) can full-fat coconut milk

1 cup (240 ml) low-sodium chicken broth

1–2 tbsp (15–30 ml) honey

3 tbsp (45 ml) coconut aminos

FOR SERVING

2 cups (372 g) cooked cauliflower rice

2 scallions, thinly sliced

Lime wedges

Chopped fresh basil

To make the lemongrass curry paste: Combine the lemongrass, shallot, chili, ginger, garlic, basil, oil, lime juice, salt and pepper in a food processor or high-speed blender. Blend until smooth. Set aside.

To make the curry: Place the oil in a large skillet over medium heat. Add the shrimp and cook in an even layer for 1 to 2 minutes on each side, or until pink. Cook in two batches, if needed. Set the shrimp aside.

Add the green beans to the skillet, sautéing for 2 minutes. Pour in the coconut milk, broth, honey and coconut aminos. Stir to combine. Add the prepared curry paste to the skillet and whisk to incorporate. Bring the curry to a boil and reduce to a simmer for 5 minutes to thicken. Add the shrimp back to the skillet and simmer for 1 minute to heat throughout.

To serve: Divide the rice into bowls and top with the curry. Garnish with scallions, lime wedges and basil.

NOTE: This is a balanced curry, but the serrano pepper is spicy. If you don't want to turn up the heat too much, omit the pepper or remove the seeds before adding it to the curry paste.

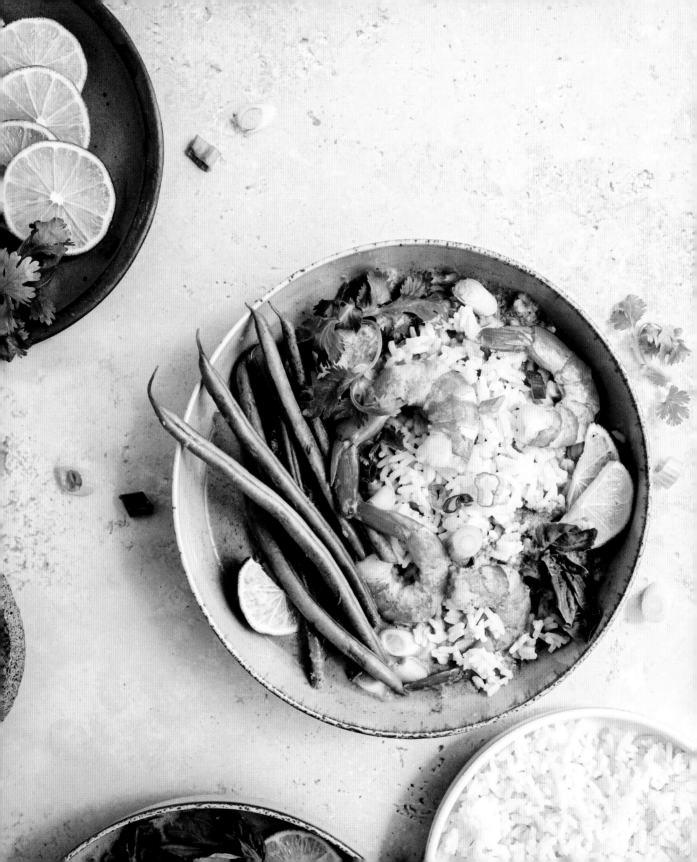

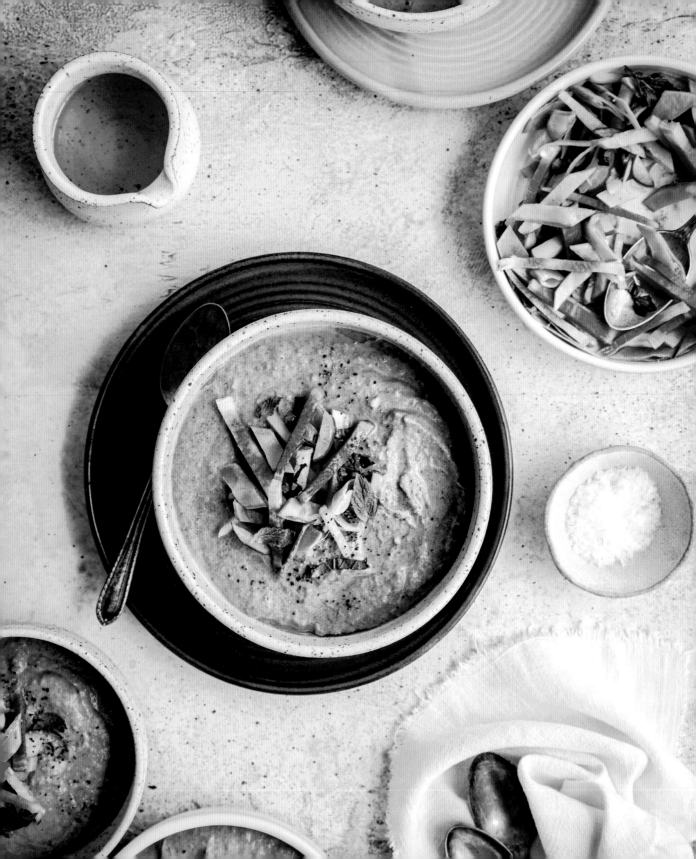

SPRING GREENS SOUP WITH PEA AND RADISH SLAW

I applaud the versatility of soup: it can be the richest comfort food or the lightest spring dinner when you're ready for longer days and shorter sleeves to make an appearance. I get a little "green happy" at the farmers' market when spring rolls around, forgetting that I don't cook with anything other than zucchini during the week. This soup is my go-to when my fridge is full of wilted greens that need to be used. I like to top my bowl off with a crunchy slaw to add some texture to the puréed soup.

Serves: 4

FOR THE SLAW

1 cup (110 g) sugar snap peas, julienned

½ cup (58 g) radishes, thinly sliced

1 tbsp (15 ml) red wine vinegar

½ tsp sea salt

1 tbsp (6 g) chopped fresh mint

FOR THE SOUP

1 tbsp (15 ml) olive oil

2 shallots, chopped

2 cloves garlic, minced

1 (2-inch [5-cm]) piece fresh ginger, grated

1 quart (960 ml) chicken bone broth

1 cup (145 g) green peas

1 cup (94 g) broccoli florets

4 cups (268 g) greens of choice, such as kale, spinach, chard, etc.

½ cup (120 ml) milk of choice (I use canned coconut milk.)

¼ cup (23 g) fresh mint

To make the slaw: Toss together the snap peas, radishes, vinegar, salt and mint. Set aside to marinate while the soup cooks.

To make the soup: Heat the oil in a large pot over medium heat. Add the shallots, garlic and ginger to the pot. Sauté for 2 to 3 minutes, until fragrant. Add the broth, peas, broccoli, greens and milk. Bring to a boil, then reduce to a simmer for 12 minutes, until the vegetables are soft and wilted.

Add the mint to the soup, then use a high-speed blender or an immersion blender to blend the soup until smooth. Serve the soup topped with slaw.

CREAMY ROASTED FENNEL CAULIFLOWER SOUP

There are few things I find more comforting than putting on a pair of cozy socks and heating up a mild-yet-flavorful bowl of soup during the long New York winters. Two years ago, I started adding roasted fennel to my soups and found it to be the perfect flavor addition that is just enough without overpowering the dish. Here I've also added roasted cauliflower and hearty bone broth. This soup can stand alone as a lunch or light dinner, or it's also a lovely complement to a larger main course.

Serves: 4 to 6

FOR THE SOUP

1 large head cauliflower, cut into florets

1 bulb fennel, halved and sliced

1 shallot, diced

3 tbsp (45 ml) olive oil, divided

1 quart (960 ml) chicken bone broth

½ cup (120 ml) canned coconut milk

2 tbsp (30 ml) lemon juice

½ tsp sea salt

½ tsp black pepper

2 cloves garlic, minced

FOR SERVING

Olive oil

Chopped fresh parsley

Croutons

Preheat the oven to 425°F (218°C). Line a baking sheet with parchment paper.

To make the soup: Toss the cauliflower, fennel and shallot with 2 tablespoons (30 ml) of the oil and place the mixture on the baking sheet. Bake for 25 minutes, until the vegetables are tender, flipping halfway through. Place the roasted veggies in a blender with the broth and blend for 2 minutes, or until smooth. Add the coconut milk, lemon juice, salt and pepper, and blend again to combine.

Add the remaining 1 tablespoon (15 ml) of oil to a saucepan over medium heat with garlic. Sauté for 2 minutes, then pour in the blended soup. Bring to a low boil and reduce to a simmer for 15 minutes to allow the soup to thicken.

To serve: Garnish with a drizzle of olive oil, fresh parsley and a thick crouton.

NOTE: I used toasted grain-free focaccia to make my croutons. Use any variety of homemade bread, toast wedges of your favorite store-bought bread, or omit if desired.

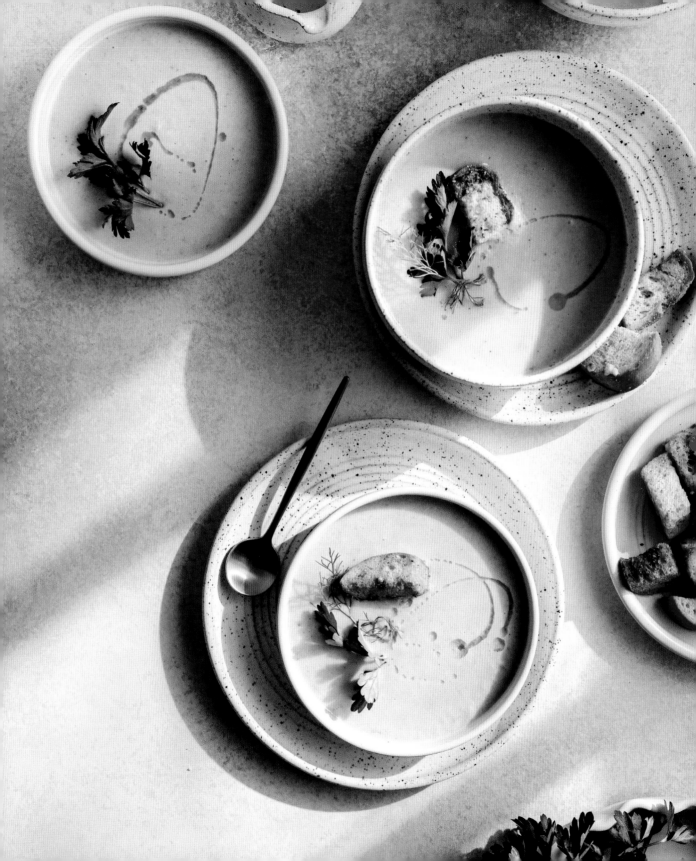

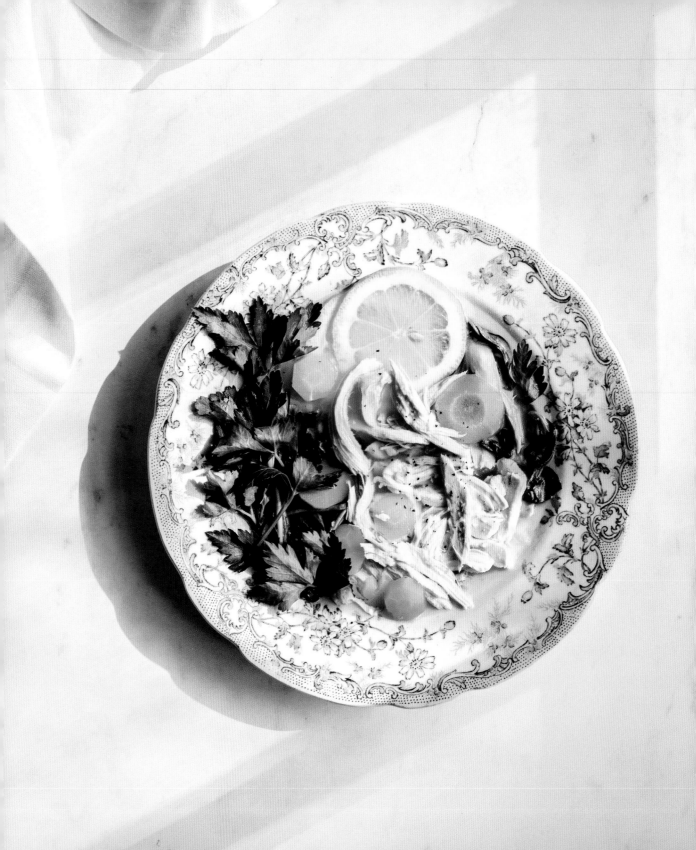

LEMON-GINGER CHICKEN SOUP

Few things embody the essence of "cozy" better than the combination of lemon, ginger and chicken broth. I like routine when it comes to cooking for myself, and this is a soup I turn to on an almost weekly basis when my body feels tired or my gut needs some extra nourishment. In the summer I'll make a "cheat" version of this with some leftover shredded chicken breasts and some bone broth, though the real version is truly easy and worth shredding a whole chicken for. Serve it with a handful of fresh herbs for maximum comfort and flavor.

Serves: 6

FOR THE SOUP

1 (4–5 lbs [1.8–2.2 kg]) whole chicken

2 shallots, peeled

2 cloves garlic, peeled

1 (2-inch [5-cm]) piece fresh ginger, peeled

1 tsp sea salt

½ tsp black pepper

Juice of 1 lemon

4 carrots, peeled and sliced

2 cups (60 g) spinach

FOR SERVING

1 cup (60 g) finely chopped fresh parsley

1 lemon, thinly sliced

To make the soup: Combine the whole chicken, shallots, garlic, ginger, salt and pepper in a large pot. Fill it with enough water to cover plus 2 inches (5 cm). Cover and bring to a boil, then reduce the heat and simmer for 1 hour, or until the chicken is cooked and tender.

Remove the chicken to a large board or plate.

Strain the broth into a large pot and return it to the heat. Add the lemon juice and carrots. Bring to a boil, then reduce to a simmer for 10 minutes, or until the carrots are tender.

Shred the chicken using a fork, discarding the bones or saving for another broth. Return the shredded chicken to the simmering pot. Add the spinach and simmer for 5 to 10 minutes, until the chicken is heated and the spinach is wilted.

To serve: Serve topped with the parsley and lemon slices.

WEEKNIGHT MEATBALL SOUP

My only qualm with soups is that many require a barrage of herbs and ample simmering time. But what if you worked late, walked the dog and then realized you already ate your leftover Thai food and need dinner in a pinch? This meatball soup is my answer for those weeknights when I just want to sip a large mug of broth by the window and then collapse onto the couch. Bonus: You can make it with whatever ground meat you have on hand!

Serves: 4

FOR THE MEATBALLS

1½ lbs (680 g) ground turkey or ground chicken

1 large egg

¼ cup (15 g) finely chopped fresh parsley

½ tsp garlic powder

½ tsp onion powder

½ tsp sea salt

¼ tsp black pepper

FOR THE SOUP

2 tbsp (30 ml) olive oil

2 cloves garlic, minced

2 shallots, thinly sliced

1 quart (960 ml) chicken bone broth

2 cups (134 g) torn kale or spinach

Grated Parmesan (optional)

To make the meatballs: Mix the turkey, egg, parsley, garlic powder, onion powder, salt and pepper. Roll into twelve small meatballs.

To make the soup: Place the oil in a large pot over medium-high heat. Add the garlic and shallots, and sauté for 2 minutes. Pour in the broth and bring to a simmer.

Carefully drop the meatballs into the soup and allow them to simmer for 18 to 20 minutes, until they are cooked through. I suggest checking with a meat thermometer to ensure they are 165°F (74°C).

Add the kale to the pot and reduce the heat to medium-low. Allow it to simmer for 5 minutes, until the kale is wilted. Divide the soup into four bowls and serve topped with grated Parmesan (if using).

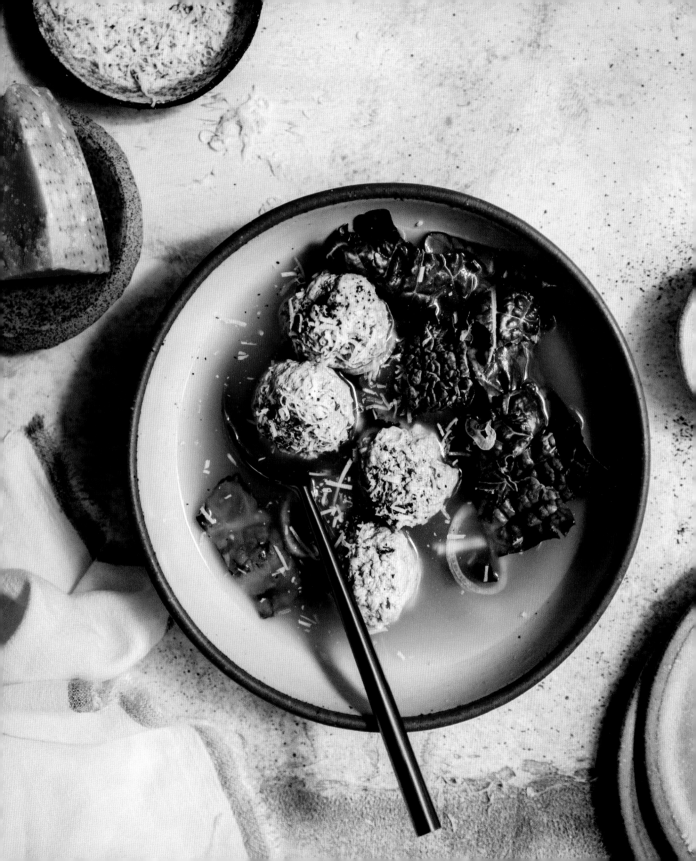

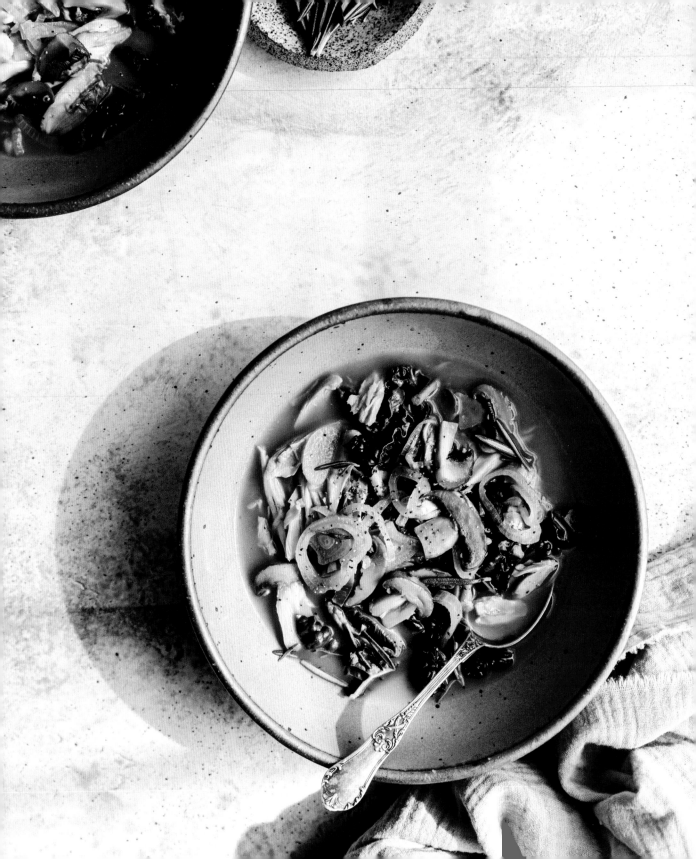

BALSAMIC CHICKEN MUSHROOM STEW

Here's a life tip for you: put balsamic vinegar in your stew. Always. Every time. No disrespect to the vinegar-less stews out there, but it adds a depth of flavor that transforms your everyday soup situation into something magical and robust. Here, the tart vinegar pairs perfectly with the savory mushrooms, which are all beautifully balanced against the salty bone broth. I like to serve stew in a wide, low bowl so there's more surface area for sprinkling the vinegar on top. It's science.

Serves: 4

2 tbsp (30 ml) olive oil

2 shallots, diced

2 cloves garlic, minced

1 lb (454 g) cremini or white mushrooms, sliced

2 tbsp (30 ml) balsamic vinegar, plus more for serving (optional)

1 lb (454 g) cooked shredded chicken (a mix of dark and light meat)

3 cups (720 ml) chicken bone broth

¼ cup (60 ml) canned coconut milk

1 tbsp (2 g) fresh rosemary

2 cups (134 g) chopped kale or spinach

½ tsp sea salt

½ tsp black pepper

Heat the oil in a large pot over medium heat. Add the shallots and garlic to the pot. Sauté for 1 to 2 minutes, until fragrant. Add the mushrooms and vinegar, and sauté for 2 to 3 minutes to caramelize. Stir in the chicken, broth, coconut milk, rosemary, kale, salt and pepper.

Bring the stew to a boil, then reduce it to a simmer for 15 minutes to thicken the broth and wilt the kale.

Serve topped with an extra drizzle of balsamic vinegar, if desired.

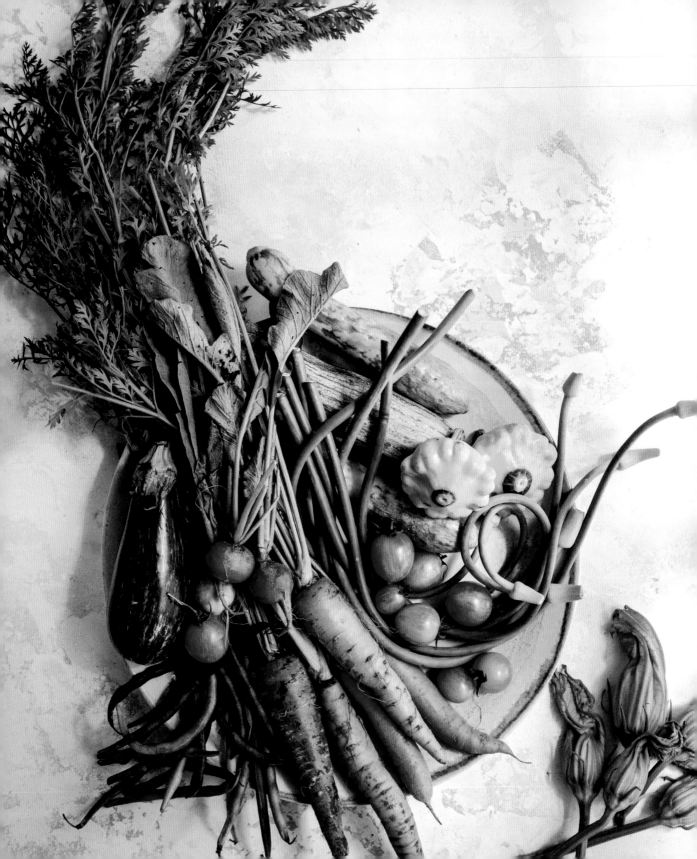

VEGETABLES AND SIDES FOR ANY OCCASION

There is nothing quite as optimistic as fresh fruits and vegetables appearing season after season, showing new faces and new colors as the temperatures drop and rise again. I'm especially drawn toward the greens and pinks that emerge in spring after a long winter, signaling new beginnings. But there is evergreen life and beauty in the flavors of every season, proving time and again that new life is always on the horizon.

Quality produce can do the work for you, so I try to do most of my shopping at farmers' markets when possible. If I'm having guests over, there's a 10/10 chance I'll be making my Smashed Potatoes with Gremolata (page 83) and my Ten-Minute Zucchini Ribbon Salad (page 91). If it's just me, my Mint and Pine Nut Sautéed Zucchini (page 76) is always on the menu.

MINT AND PINE NUT SAUTÉED ZUCCHINI

I'm a serial monogamist with my food, it's true. When I find something good that works, I commit one-hundred-percent to a long-term relationship that involves cooking it every single night. My current fling is zucchini, and we've been steady for about two years now. Each week I haul about four pounds (1.8 kg) the of zucchini up several city blocks and jam them all in my tiny fridge, just to roast them quite unceremoniously. Zucchini is a great vehicle for herbs, citrus and toasted nuts, so this is the recipe I turn to when I want a little variety.

Serves: 4 to 6

¼ cup (35 g) pine nuts

2 tbsp (30 ml) olive or coconut oil

1 shallot, thinly sliced

1 lb (454 g) zucchini and/or yellow squash, sliced into ¼-inch (6-mm) pieces

¼ cup (23 g) chopped mint

½ tsp Maldon sea salt

Heat a large skillet over medium-high heat. Add the pine nuts and sauté for 2 minutes to lightly toast. Set aside.

Add the oil and shallot to the skillet. Sauté for 2 minutes. Add the zucchini and sauté for 8 minutes, or until softened while still crisp on the edges. Arrange the squash on a platter and top with toasted pine nuts, mint and salt.

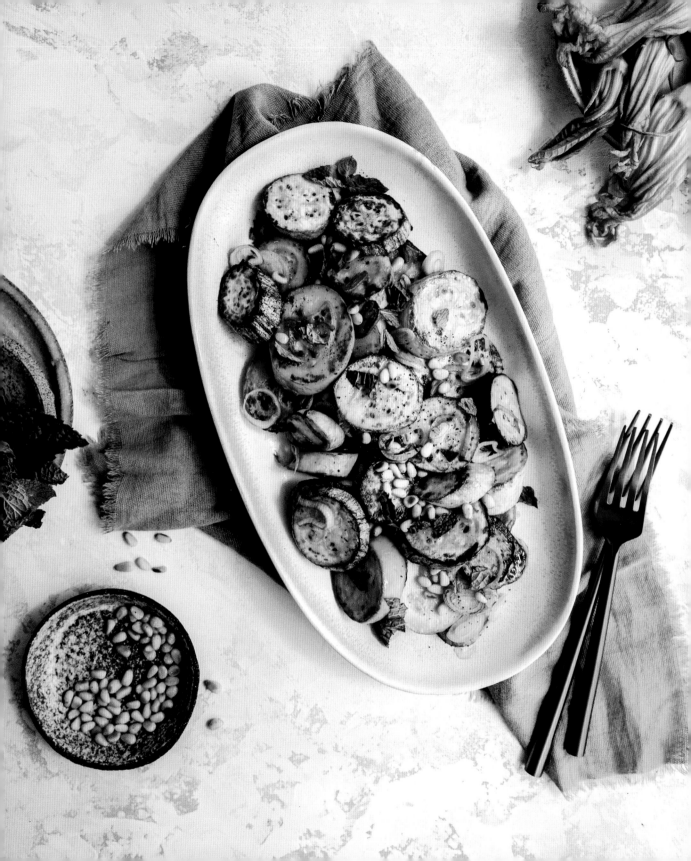

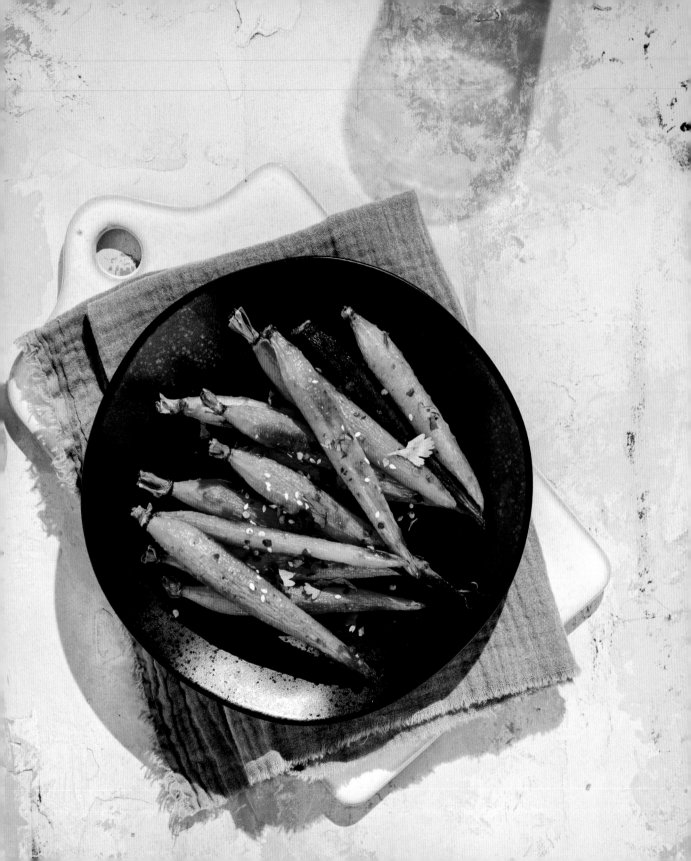

SWEET AND SPICY ROASTED CARROTS

One key truth I've learned throughout my creative career is that inspiration doesn't come from billboards. Sometimes it's found in wildflowers or a bunch of brightly colored carrots. It comes in whispers, and it grows louder when you pick it up and get to work, but it rarely shouts. It's in the curious effort to be inspired that we end up finding ourselves with new ideas. And that's often my process for creating a recipe; these unassuming yet boldly flavored carrots are no exception. They're the result of curiosity and experimentation, and they're wildly addictive.

Serves: 4

2 lbs (907 g) carrots, peeled

3 tbsp (45 ml) olive oil

2 tbsp (30 ml) honey or maple syrup

2 tsp (6 g) harissa paste

½ tsp sea salt

¼ tsp black pepper

Pinch of red pepper flakes (optional)

1 tbsp (9 g) sesame seeds

2 tbsp (6 g) finely chopped fresh cilantro

Preheat the oven to 400°F (204°C).

Arrange the carrots on a baking sheet so that they are not touching. You want them separated enough to get crispy; use two pans, if needed.

Stir together the oil, honey, harissa, salt and pepper. Drizzle the mixture evenly over the carrots and roast for 35 to 40 minutes, flipping halfway through.

Top the carrots with red pepper flakes (if using), sesame seeds and cilantro.

ROOT VEGETABLE AGRODOLCE

I first encountered agrodolce on a restaurant client shoot and was intrigued by the name alone. It's a sweet-and-sour Italian sauce that I've now added to the list of reasons I wish I had been born in Italy. There's hardly a food on the planet that I wouldn't eat smothered in agrodolce, but here I've paired it with some approachable root vegetables to help ease you into my agrodolce cult.

Serves: 4

FOR THE VEGETABLES

2–3 large beets (I use one golden and one red.)

6 large carrots, peeled and roughly chopped

2 sweet potatoes, sliced into half moons about 1-inch (2.5-cm) thick (I use a purple sweet potato and a regular yam.)

1 delicata squash, sliced in half lengthwise and sliced into half moons

2 shallots, quartered

2 tbsp (30 ml) olive oil

½ tsp sea salt

½ tsp black pepper

FOR THE AGRODOLCE

½ cup (120 ml) apple cider vinegar

¼ cup (60 ml) maple syrup

½ tsp sea salt

½ tsp red pepper flakes (optional)

FOR SERVING

Fresh thyme

Maldon sea salt

Preheat the oven to 425°F (218°C). Line a baking sheet with parchment paper.

To make the vegetables: Wrap the beets in a large piece of tinfoil and place them on the end of the baking sheet. Toss the carrots, sweet potatoes, squash and shallots with oil, salt and pepper. Spread the vegetables evenly on the baking sheet and place it in the oven for 35 to 40 minutes, stirring halfway through. The vegetables should be crispy and the beets should be fork-tender.

Unwrap the beets and rinse under cool water to peel. Cut them into quarters and toss with the roasted vegetables on a platter.

While the vegetables are roasting, make the agrodolce: Combine the vinegar, maple syrup, salt and red pepper flakes (if using) in a saucepan over medium heat. Bring to a boil, then reduce to a simmer for about 10 minutes, or until the sauce is thickened.

To serve: Pour the agrodolce over the vegetables to coat. Serve topped with fresh thyme and flakey salt.

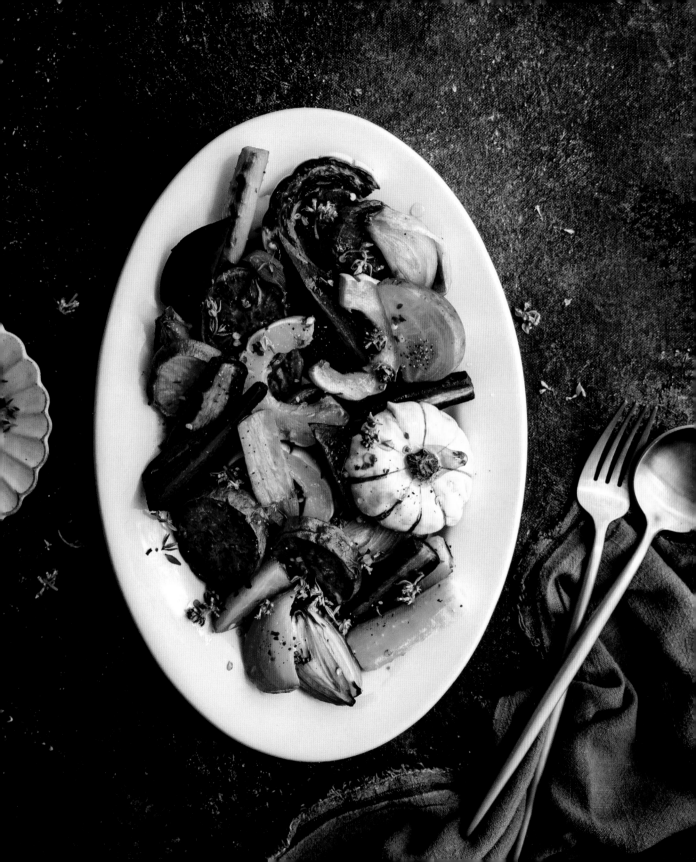

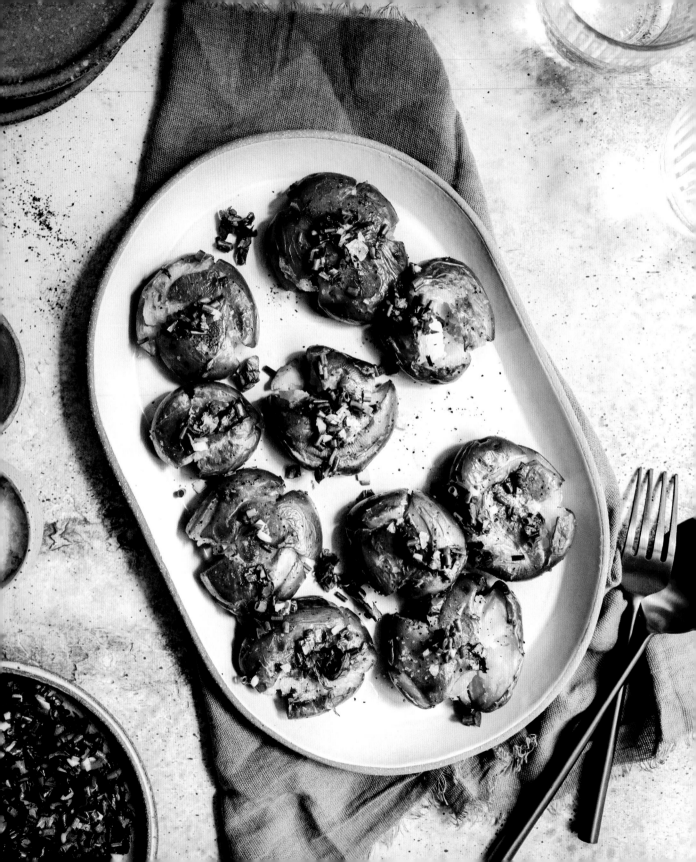

SMASHED POTATOES WITH GREMOLATA

Let's cut to the chase: gremolata is the bomb-dot-com, so much so that it renders these delightful crispy potatoes as a mere vehicle for the gremolata goodness—which is saying something, because smashed potatoes are the greatest thing to happen to the spud industry since french fries. I like to add chives to my gremolata for an extra herby punch, though you could use whatever herbs you have on hand and you'd still be winning. The potatoes have the tender deliciousness of a baked potato with the crunchy integrity of a fry. It's a dream-team combo that'll please any crowd.

Serves: 6

FOR THE POTATOES

2 lbs (907 g) baby Yukon gold potatoes

2 tbsp (30 ml) olive oil

½ tsp sea salt

¼ tsp black pepper

½ tsp onion powder

FOR THE GREMOLATA

1 cup (60 g) finely chopped fresh flat-leaf parsley

⅓ cup (18 g) chopped fresh chives

2 cloves garlic, minced

Juice of ½ lemon

⅓ cup (79 ml) olive oil

½ tsp sea salt

Preheat the oven to 425°F (218°C). Line a large baking sheet with tinfoil.

To make the potatoes: Place the potatoes in a large pot and cover by 1 inch (2.5 cm) of water. Bring the water to a boil, then reduce to a simmer for 12 to 15 minutes, or until the potatoes are softened. Drain the potatoes and place them on the prepared baking sheet.

Use the bottom of a mug or glass to smash the potatoes, then toss them with the oil, salt, pepper and onion powder. Bake for 25 to 30 minutes, flipping halfway through. The potatoes should be crispy and golden when finished.

To make the gremolata: Stir together the parsley, chives, garlic, lemon juice, oil and salt in a small bowl.

Serve the gremolata over the crispy potatoes.

PEACH AND HEIRLOOM TOMATO PANZANELLA

The low-key joy of summer is perfectly encapsulated by this bright, fresh riff on the classic bread salad. Sweet peaches, crunchy croutons, ripe tomatoes and a zesty dressing combine to make a harmonious, flavorful dish. Preheat the grill, add some chicken or fish and you've got an ideal summer meal waiting to happen.

Serves: 4

6 slices grain-free bread, cubed

3 tbsp (45 ml) olive oil, divided

2 tbsp (30 ml) balsamic vinegar

4 cups (80 g) arugula

4 peaches, thinly sliced

2 large heirloom tomatoes, sliced

½ cup (75 g) heirloom cherry tomatoes, halved

1 tomatillo, thinly sliced

¼ cup (8 g) roughly torn fresh basil

½ tsp sea salt

½ tsp black pepper

1 burrata ball, roughly torn

Preheat the oven to 375°F (190°C).

Toss together the bread and 1 tablespoon (15 ml) of the oil, and spread it evenly on a baking sheet. Toast the bread for 8 to 10 minutes, or until golden. Set the bread aside to cool.

Whisk together the vinegar and the remaining 2 tablespoons (30 ml) of oil. Arrange the arugula, peaches, tomatoes and tomatillo on a platter. Drizzle the salad with the vinegar mixture, tossing to coat evenly. Sprinkle the basil, salt and pepper evenly over the salad.

Top with the burrata and toasted croutons, and serve immediately.

NOTE: If you're waiting a few hours before serving, hold off on topping the salad with the dressing, burrata and croutons to prevent sogginess.

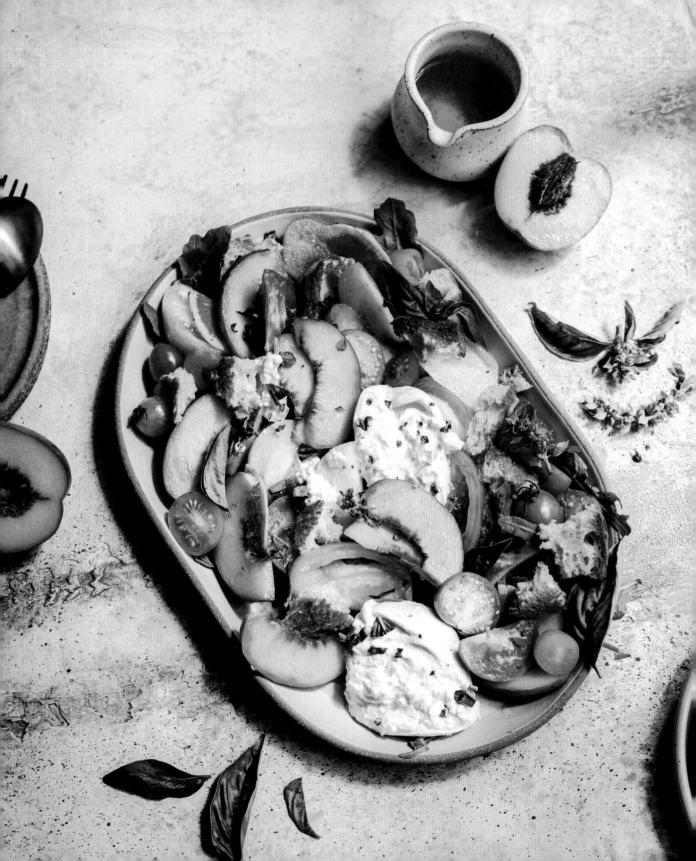

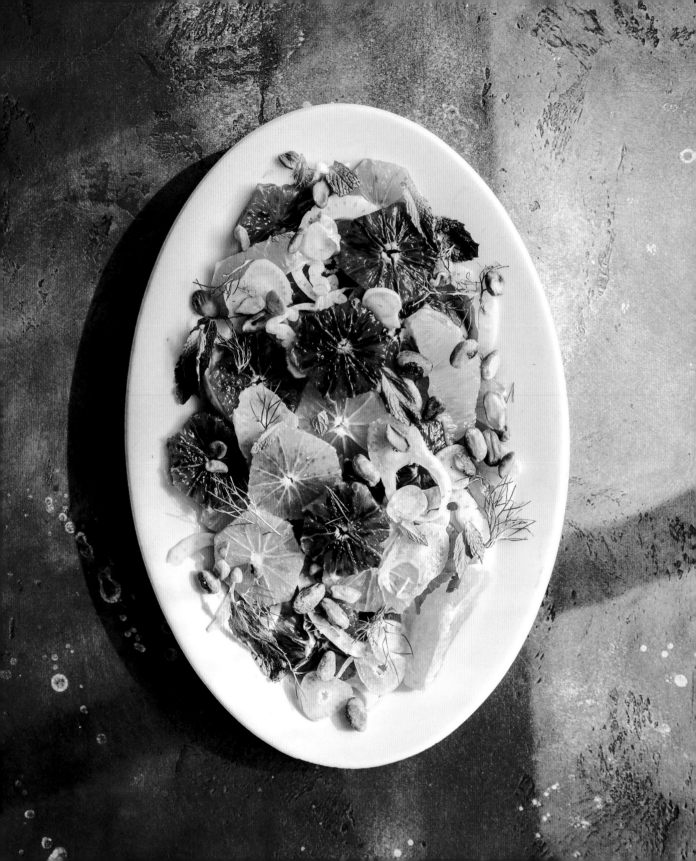

BLOOD ORANGE AND FENNEL SALAD

I just love that blood orange season is in the middle of winter. Something about it seems so counterintuitive to the rest of what is in season during that time of year. It's unexpectedly light and sweet, and it contrasts so beautifully against the stinging cold and the rich winter food. This salad is a celebration of all the wonders of winter citrus with juicy oranges on a backdrop of crisp fennel, fresh mint and crunchy pistachios.

Serves: 4

4 blood oranges

1 medium navel orange

1 small fennel bulb

Juice of 1 lemon

2 tsp (10 ml) honey

2 tbsp (30 ml) olive oil

¼ cup (31 g) pistachios

¼ cup (23 g) fresh mint

1 tsp Maldon sea salt

Peel and slice the blood oranges crosswise in thin slices, then peel and segment the navel orange, removing the white pith.

Use a mandolin or a sharp knife to shave the fennel bulb into very thin slices. Arrange the fennel on a platter with the orange slices and segments.

In a small bowl, whisk together the lemon juice, honey and oil. Scatter the pistachios and mint over the salad. Drizzle with the lemon dressing and sprinkle the salad with flakey salt. Serve immediately.

LEMON-ARTICHOKE PESTO PASTA

There are certain streets in New York where everything smells like an Italian feast waiting to be enjoyed. It's hard to run a single errand without having to walk down one of these streets, so I'm basically walking around in a constant state of hangry. The cure? Pesto pasta with tender artichokes. It's a quick-fix packed with flavor that doesn't require hours of cooking heat, which is my kind of dish.

Serves: 4

½ lb (227 g) cassava flour spaghetti or similar gluten-free pasta

2 tbsp (30 ml) olive oil

2 shallots, finely chopped

2 cups (134 g) Tuscan kale, roughly chopped

1 (14-oz [400-g]) can artichoke hearts, drained

Juice of 1 lemon

1 cup (260 g) pesto of choice (page 130)

Zest of 1 lemon, for topping

Maldon sea salt, for topping

Bring a large pot of water to a boil with a pinch of salt. Add the spaghetti and cook according to the package until al dente. While the pasta boils, heat the oil in a medium-sized skillet over medium heat. Add the shallots and sauté for 2 minutes. Add the kale and artichoke hearts, and sauté to warm and wilt the kale.

Drain the cooked spaghetti and add it to the skillet, stirring to mix it with the artichoke hearts and kale. Turn off heat and stir in the lemon juice and pesto.

Divide the pasta among four plates. Top with lemon zest and flakey salt.

NOTE: This dish goes great with some shrimp or roasted chicken added for protein.

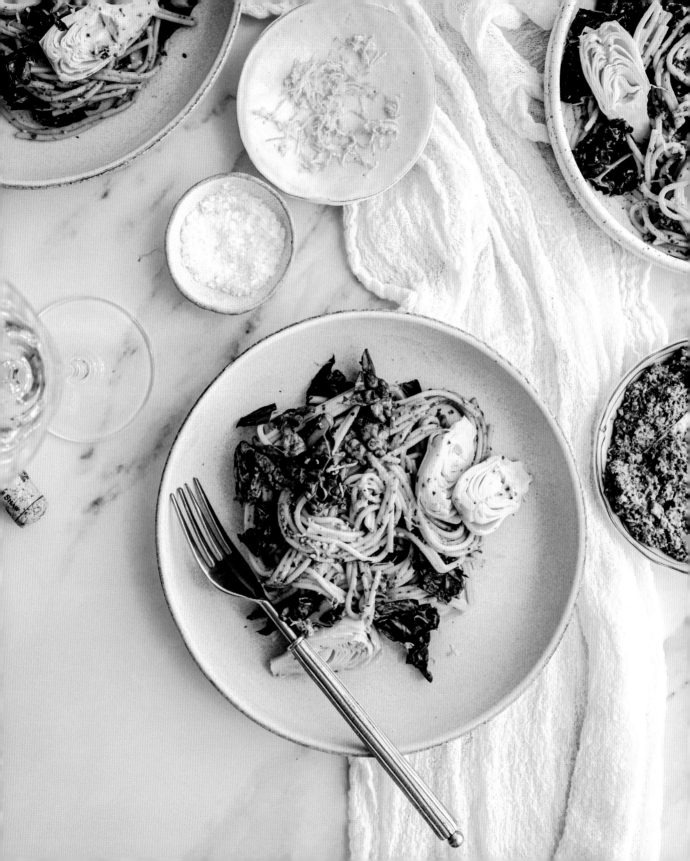

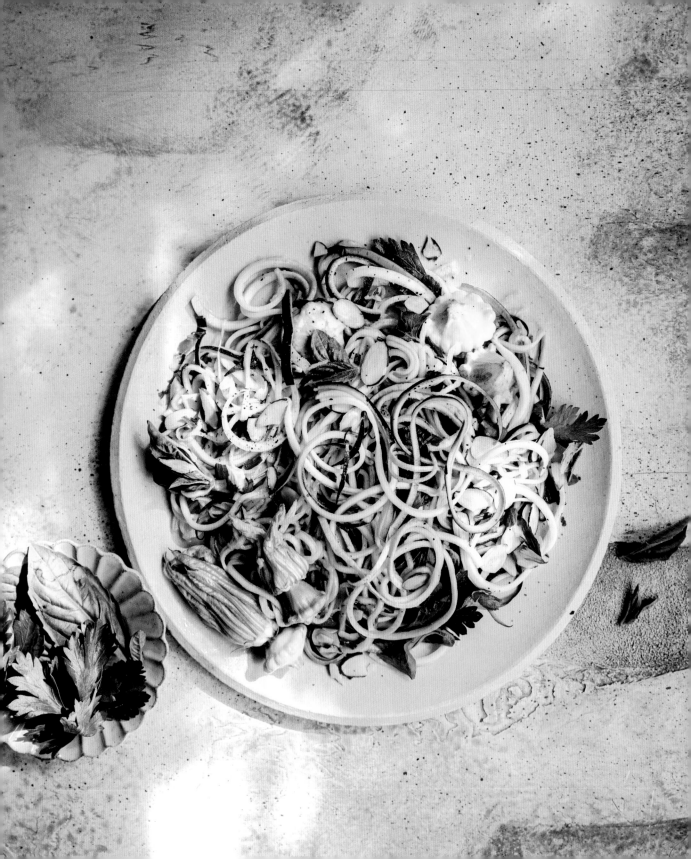

TEN-MINUTE ZUCCHINI RIBBON SALAD

People in my line of work are known to overthink. It comes with creative jobs along with the mood boards and sketchbooks, and it sticks with you throughout your career and into your personal life. It's a daily practice to get my mind to quiet, even for a little while. I think I like cooking with zucchini so much because I can do it with a bit of reckless abandon: No recipe or notes. No deep concentration or second-guessing. Just some off-key singing to Coldplay while I add pinches of salt or squeezes of lemon. And it's delicious every time. Zucchini just kinda goes with the flow.

Serves: 4

1 lb (454 g) zucchini, spiralized or shaved with a peeler

Juice of 1 lemon

2 tsp (10 ml) honey

1 tbsp (15 ml) olive oil

½ tsp sea salt

½ tsp black pepper

¼ cup (8 g) torn fresh basil

¼ cup (15 g) finely chopped fresh parsley

2–3 squash blossoms, for garnish

Arrange the zucchini noodles on a serving plate. In a small bowl, whisk together the lemon juice, honey, oil, salt and pepper.

Drizzle the dressing evenly over the zucchini and toss to coat. Stir in the basil and parsley, then top the zucchini with squash blossoms.

NOTE: If you have a spiralizer with multiple blades, I like to make the squashes a few different sizes to make the dish more visually interesting. I also like to use a mix of yellow and green squashes for a more dynamic color story.

DUKKAH ROASTED EGGPLANTS AND WHIPPED TAHINI

There has always been a specific creative energy bubbling inside of me that shows its best side on two different occasions: when I'm photographing in a restaurant and when I'm styling a savory dish that involves intricate, beautiful vegetables. There's something about the colors and the organic shapes and textures that just gives me endless ideas. This dish is a feat of both flavor and presentation. The whipped tahini, coarse dukkah and fresh herbs make this simple dish look like a work of art, and they're also a flavor combo to rule them all.

Serves: 4 to 6

FOR THE EGGPLANTS

4 small eggplants

1 tbsp (15 ml) olive oil

½ tsp sea salt

FOR THE ALMOND DUKKAH

⅓ cup (48 g) almonds

¼ cup (31 g) pistachios

2 tbsp (18 g) sesame seeds

2 tsp (2 g) ground coriander

2 tsp (2 g) ground cumin

½ tsp sea salt

¼ tsp black pepper

FOR THE WHIPPED TAHINI

½ cup (120 ml) smooth tahini

1 clove garlic, minced

1 tbsp (15 ml) lemon juice

½ tsp sea salt

⅓ cup (79 ml) cold water

FOR SERVING

Finely chopped fresh mint or cilantro

Preheat the oven to 350°F (177°C).

To make the eggplants: Slice the eggplants in half lengthwise, then use a sharp knife to cut a thin score into the flesh of the eggplants in a crosshatch pattern. Place the eggplants cut side up on a baking sheet and drizzle evenly with oil and salt. Bake for 45 minutes, or until the eggplants are tender.

While the eggplants cook, make the almond dukkah: Place the almonds, pistachios, sesame seeds, coriander, cumin, salt and pepper in a food processor. Pulse for a few seconds until a coarse mixture is formed. Pour into a bowl and set aside.

To make the whipped tahini: Combine the tahini, garlic, lemon and salt in a blender or food processor. Blend until smooth. With the blender running, slowly drizzle in cold water until emulsified and lighter in color.

Top the roasted eggplant with whipped tahini. Dust with a sprinkle of dukkah and mint.

NOTE: I used small graffiti eggplants, but whatever you have available will do!

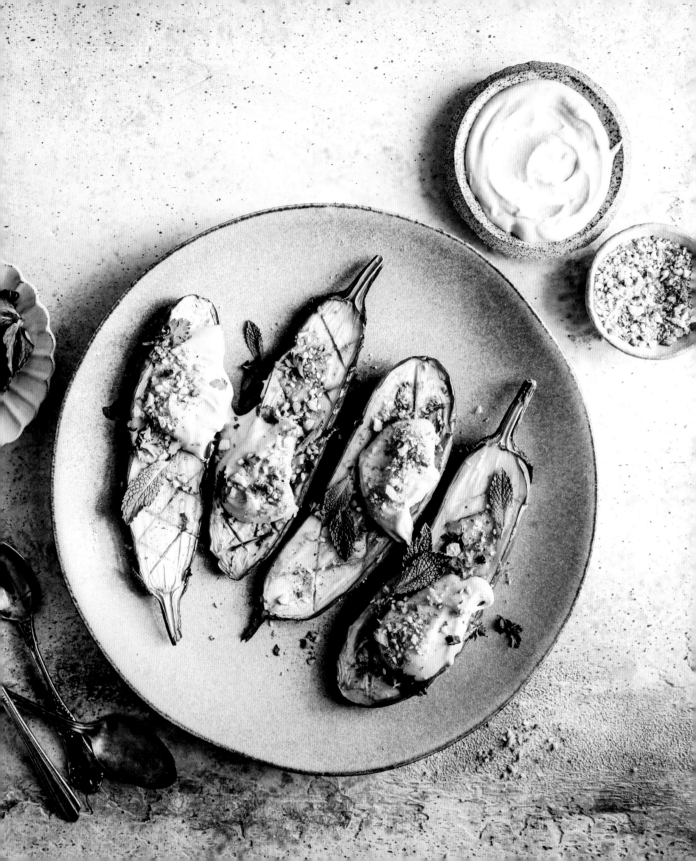

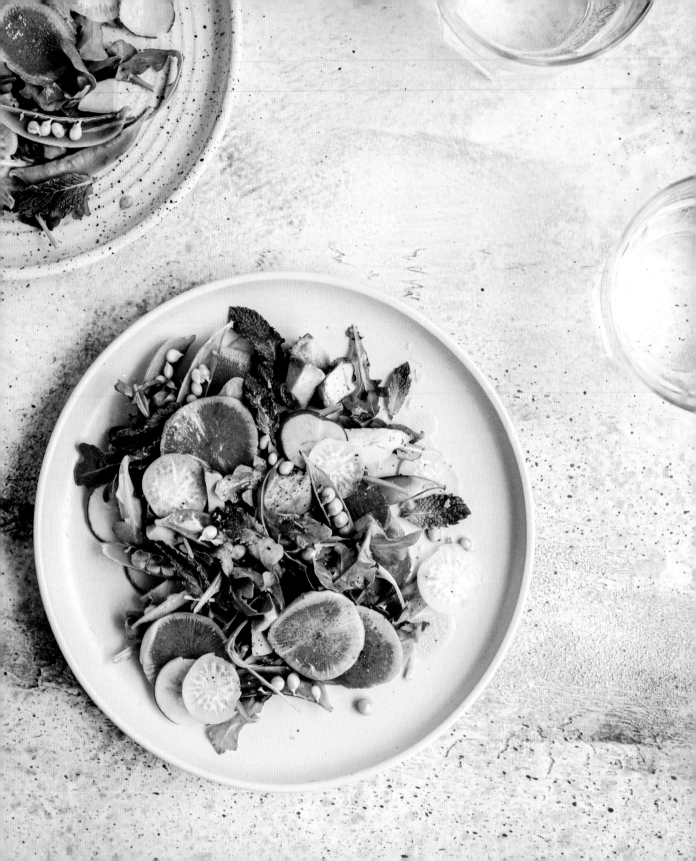

SPRING PEA AND RADISH SALAD WITH MINT

I remember the first day of spring I ever experienced after moving to New York: It was beautiful in a way you can experience only in Manhattan. The Village was lined with white blossom trees and Washington Square Park's fountain was turned on for the first time after the snowy winter. The park benches were crowded with hundreds of conversations. And I walked through it all to the farmers' market where I found tables covered in radishes—the unassuming kinds that burst into a million colors when you cut into them. If you thought radishes were just a garnish, think again! They're wonderful when thinly shaved with a mandolin, and they add a great contrasting crunch to a spring salad.

Serves: 4

FOR THE SALAD

4 cups (80 g) arugula

2 cups (220 g) sugar snap peas, trimmed

6–8 small radishes, thinly sliced

1 medium avocado, halved, seeded and peeled

¼ cup (26 g) packed fresh mint

FOR THE LEMON VINAIGRETTE

¼ cup (60 ml) olive oil

2 tbsp (30 ml) fresh lemon juice

Zest of ½ lemon

1 tbsp (15 ml) honey

2 tsp (10 ml) apple cider vinegar

1 tsp Dijon mustard

½ tsp sea salt

To make the salad: On a large platter, toss together the arugula, snap peas and radishes. Dice the avocado and mix it into the salad, then scatter mint leaves on top.

To make the lemon vinaigrette: In a small jar with a lid, add the oil, lemon juice, lemon zest, honey, vinegar, mustard and salt. Cover and shake to combine.

Drizzle the dressing over the salad and serve immediately.

NOTE: If you are making this salad ahead, wait until just before serving to dice the avocado and top with the dressing.

LEMONY POTATO AND GREEN BEAN SALAD

No one likes the hassle of finding a side dish to bring to a gathering or cookout. That's where this potato and green bean salad comes in. And before you write me off for being basic and predictable, this isn't the average soggy potato salad of your childhood coming back to haunt you. It's fresh, zesty, crunchy, dusted with fresh herbs and aesthetically pleasing AF. Go ahead and propose a salad competition at your next family barbecue, because you've got this one in the bag.

Serves: 4 to 6

FOR THE SALAD

1 lb (454 g) mini Yukon gold potatoes

2 cups (220 g) thin green beans, ends trimmed

2 small radishes, thinly sliced

Juice of 1 lemon

3 tbsp (45 ml) olive oil

1 tbsp (15 ml) champagne vinegar

½ tsp sea salt

½ tsp black pepper

FOR SERVING

4 hard boiled eggs, halved

½ cup (90 g) green olives

¼ cup (12 g) chopped fresh chives

2 tbsp (7 g) chopped fresh dill

To make the salad: Place the potatoes in a large pot of water and bring to a boil. Cook for 8 minutes, or until fork-tender. Remove the potatoes—leaving the water in the pot—and set aside to cool, then slice into halves.

While the potatoes cool, return the pot to the stove and add the green beans. Boil for 2 to 3 minutes, then drain and quickly blanch with cold water. Add them to a platter or serving bowl with the potatoes and radishes.

Stir together the lemon juice, oil, vinegar, salt and pepper until well combined. Drizzle the dressing over the potatoes and green beans, and toss to coat evenly.

To serve: Arrange the eggs on the platter and scatter olives, chives and dill over the top.

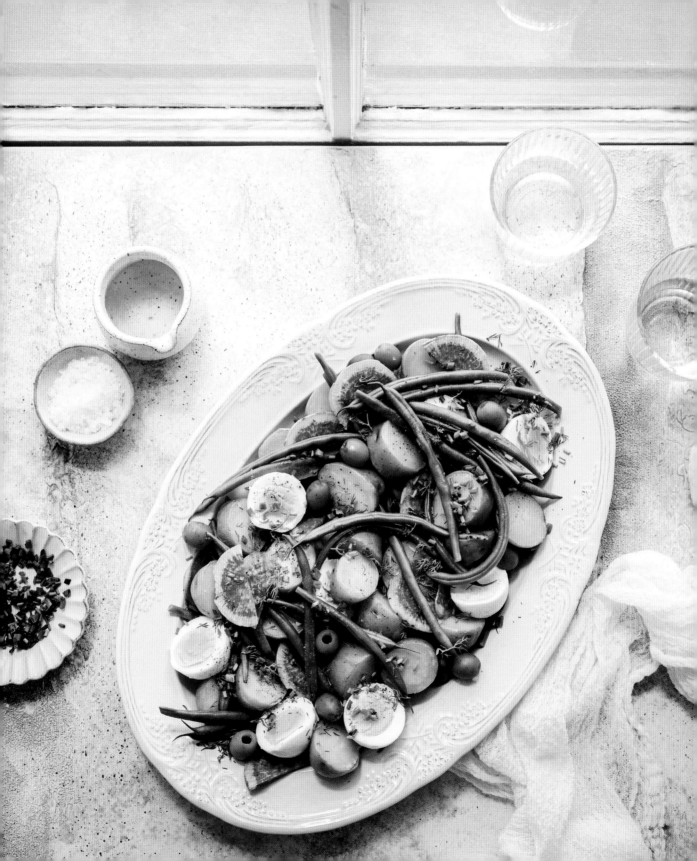

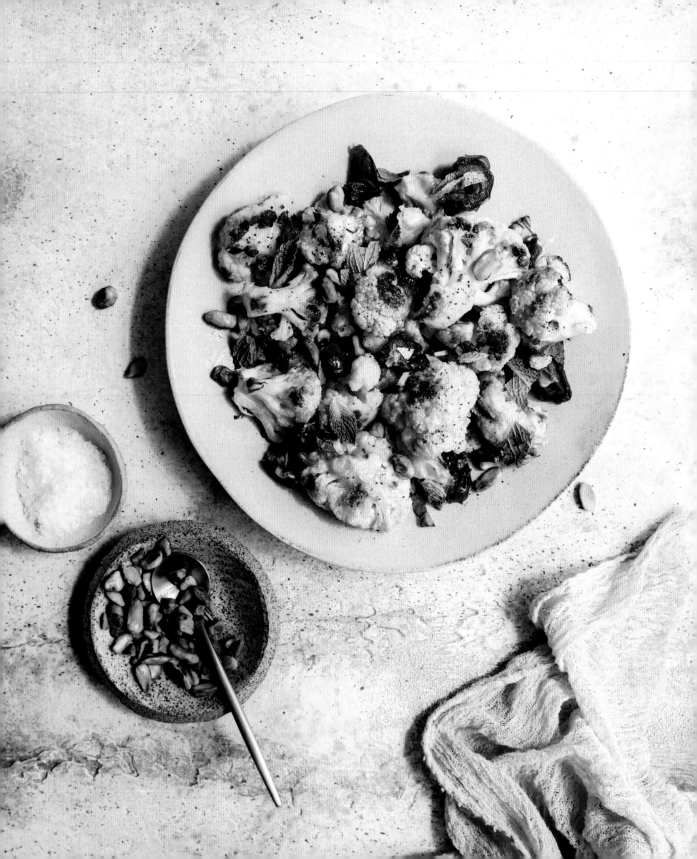

TAHINI CAULIFLOWER WITH MINT AND DATES

Tahini cauliflower is a staple "fancy food" in my family. I'll never forget the first time we all stuck our forks into a plate of the nutty deliciousness, looking at each other with wide eyes like we had struck gold. This dish is always on the list when there's a special dinner being made, no matter the occasion or main dish. We've modified the recipe over the years as we've tried new things and learned new flavor combinations. This is by far my favorite, with sweet medjool dates, fresh mint and crunchy pistachios.

Serves: 4

FOR THE SALAD

1 large head cauliflower, cut into florets

2 tbsp (30 ml) olive oil

½ tsp Maldon sea salt

¼ tsp black pepper

1 clove garlic, minced

¼ cup (60 ml) tahini

1 tsp harissa paste

1 tbsp (15 ml) lemon juice

FOR SERVING

3 medjool dates, roughly chopped

3 tbsp (18 g) chopped fresh mint

2 tbsp (15 g) pistachios

Preheat the oven to 425°F (218°C).

To make the salad: Toss the cauliflower on a large baking sheet with the oil, salt, pepper and garlic. Arrange it in an even layer. Roast the cauliflower for 25 to 30 minutes, tossing halfway through, until caramelized and golden.

While the cauliflower roasts, whisk together the tahini, harissa and lemon juice. Toss the roasted cauliflower in the tahini sauce to coat evenly.

To serve: Plate the cauliflower and top with dates, mint and pistachios. Serve immediately.

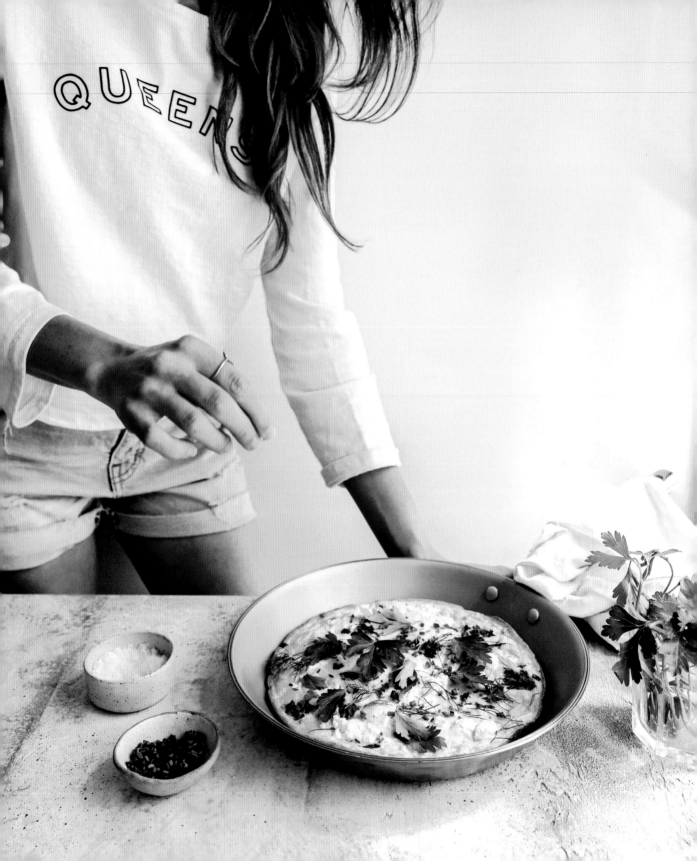

GOOD MORNINGS

If we sat down for brunch together, I don't think I'd know where to begin. Because the time it takes to eat a frittata isn't at all enough time to tell you the roller coaster I've been on as I've learned over and over what a gift it is to create and share and repeat. So instead, I'd probably let you do the talking while I sipped my coffee and looked through the windows at the golden morning. And I'd probably remark how much I love the optimism in breakfast: the fueling for a day ahead with coffee in hand. Being an artist—or hey, even being *human*—requires an embrace of discomfort, so thank goodness we have breakfast to balance it all out.

Speaking of optimism, my Butternut Shakshuka (page 102) always helps me start the day on the right foot, though I'm also especially partial to my Sweet Potato Wedges with Lemony Crushed Peas (page 109). I hope each meal in this chapter helps bring you as many good mornings as they have brought to me.

BUTTERNUT SHAKSHUKA

I first encountered shakshuka in the aptly-named "Shuka" in New York City, and it's since become my favorite brunch food. There's something so serendipitous about eggs cooked in a rich tomato sauce that just about every culture has its own version of it. I've become partial to the spice and flavor of the Middle Eastern/North African shakshuka; I like to add a touch of harissa, a Tunisian chili paste, to round out the spice. My version also includes butternut squash, which makes the dish heartier for those on a strict-Paleo diet who aren't eating the dish with bread.

Serves: 4

SHAKSHUKA

2 tbsp (30 ml) extra virgin olive oil

2 cloves garlic, minced

2 cups (410 g) diced butternut squash

½ small yellow onion, thinly sliced

1 red bell pepper, thinly sliced

1 (28-oz [793-g]) can diced tomatoes with liquid

2 tbsp (32 g) harissa paste

2 tsp (4 g) paprika

1 tsp ground cumin

½ tsp chili powder

4 large eggs

½ cup (75 g) feta (optional)

½ cup (30 g) finely chopped fresh cilantro

½ cup (30 g) finely chopped fresh parsley

Sea salt and black pepper

FOR SERVING

Toasted grain-free bread (optional)

Preheat the oven to 350°F (177°C).

To make shakshuka: Place the oil in a large oven-safe skillet over medium-high heat. Add the garlic, squash, onion and bell pepper. Sauté for about 8 minutes, or until the vegetables are soft. Add the tomatoes along with the harissa, paprika, cumin and chili powder. Stir and simmer for about 8 minutes, or until the sauce is thickened.

Make four divots in the sauce and crack an egg into each. Place the skillet in the oven and bake for 10 to 12 minutes, or until the egg whites are solid but the yolks are still runny.

Sprinkle with feta (if using), cilantro, parsley, salt and pepper.

To serve: This dish is best served immediately with toasted bread, if desired.

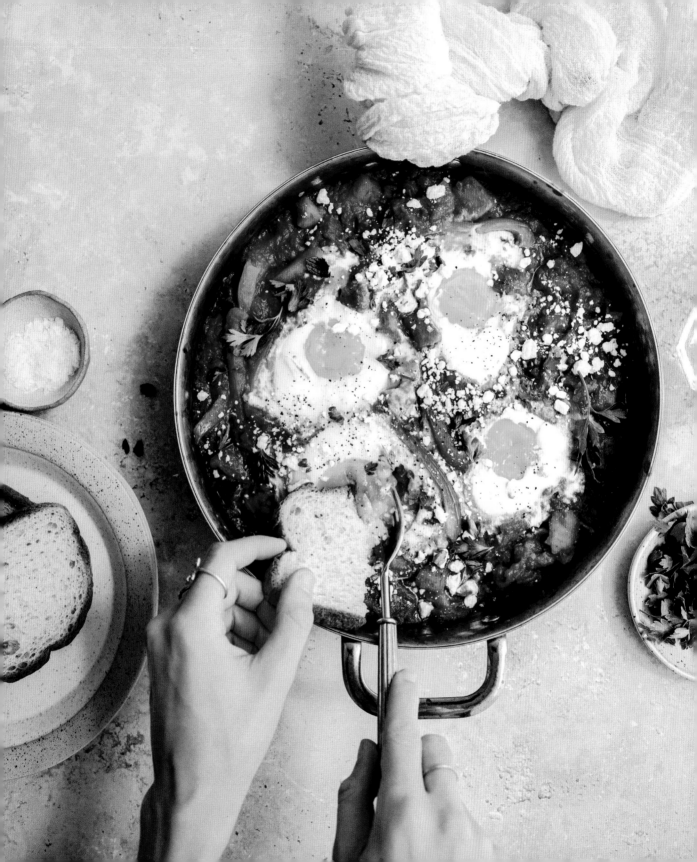

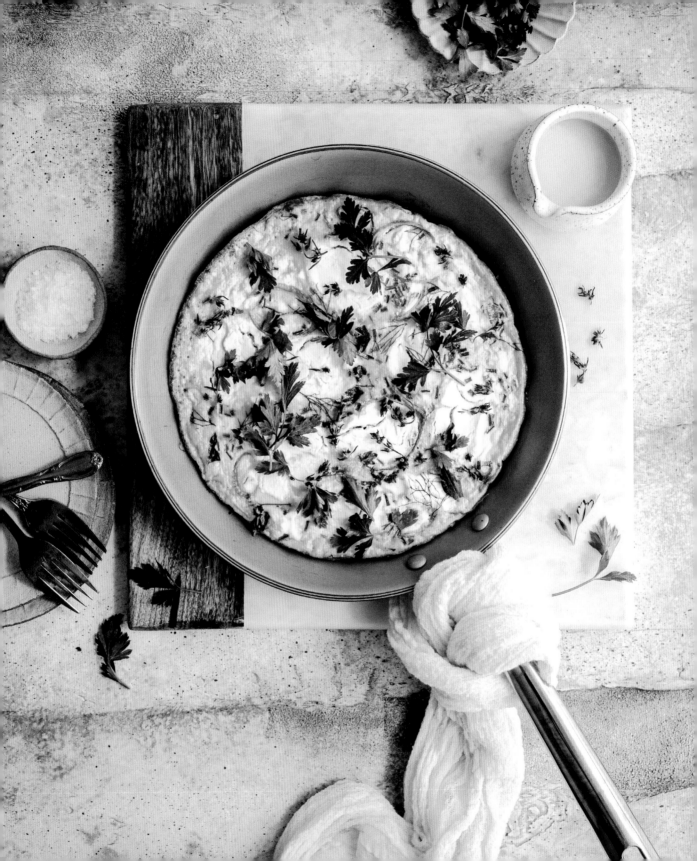

HERBY FENNEL CRUSTLESS QUICHE

Crustless quiche is a fixture in my life that began the week I discovered I have celiac disease. It was the first thing I figured out how to meal prep that I found I genuinely enjoyed eating reheated throughout the week, and it was always an easy win in the kitchen. Quiches are also a great way to be creative with your cooking since you can use any combination of meat, vegetables, cheese or even fruit that you'd like! I keep it simple with a symphony of herbs and thinly sliced fennel. Goat cheese adds a delightful touch of creaminess to this dish if you're able to tolerate dairy.

Serves: 4 to 5

1 tbsp (15 ml) avocado oil

2 cloves garlic, minced

1 bulb fennel, sliced

10 eggs

1 cup (240 ml) coconut or almond milk

¼ cup (15 g) minced fresh parsley

2 tbsp (6 g) chopped fresh chives

2 tbsp (7 g) minced fresh dill

½ tsp sea salt

¼ cup (38 g) goat cheese (optional)

Extra herbs of choice, for topping

Preheat the oven to 350°F (177°C).

Place the oil in a large, oven-safe skillet over medium heat. Add the garlic and fennel to the skillet. Sauté for 4 to 5 minutes, until the vegetables are tender.

In a medium-sized bowl, whisk together the eggs, milk, parsley, chives, dill and salt.

Pour the eggs into the skillet over the fennel. Crumble the goat cheese (if using) on top.

Continue to cook on the stovetop for 5 minutes, then place the skillet in the preheated oven and bake for 20 minutes, or until the egg mixture is set.

Serve topped with any herbs you'd like.

OLIVE OIL–BLUEBERRY BREAKFAST CAKE

Let's straighten two things out: First, I hate baking. I do it for you, and for people I love, but it is not a good time for me. Flour gets everywhere. The measuring cups have to be cleaned. And the reward isn't worth it. Second, I love blueberries so much that I'm willing to disregard the former in order to bake with them. Or rather, eat something that was baked with them. If you ever catch me with a mixing bowl and an apron, this blueberry breakfast cake is probably what's happening.

Serves: 10

Juice of ½ lemon

½ cup (120 ml) canned coconut milk

2 large eggs

¾ cup (191 g) sweet potato purée

¾ cup (150 g) coconut sugar

⅓ cup (80 ml) olive oil

1 tsp vanilla extract

1 tsp baking soda

½ tsp cream of tartar

½ tsp sea salt

1¼ cups plus 1 tbsp (170 g) cassava flour, divided

¼ cup (30 g) tapioca starch

2 tbsp (14 g) coconut flour

1 cup (148 g) fresh blueberries

Preheat the oven to 350°F (177°C). Line an 8-inch (20-cm) round baking pan with parchment paper and grease with coconut oil.

In a small bowl, stir the lemon juice into the coconut milk. Set aside.

Put the eggs, sweet potato, sugar, oil and vanilla in a blender. Blend for about 30 seconds, until smooth. Empty the mixture into a mixing bowl and stir in the baking soda, cream of tartar and salt. Pour in the coconut milk mixture and stir to combine.

Add 1¼ cups (162 g) of the cassava flour, tapioca starch and coconut flour to the bowl. Stir to combine. Toss the blueberries with the remaining 1 tablespoon (8 g) of cassava flour to lightly dust, discarding any extra flour that doesn't stick to the berries.

Fold two-thirds of the dusted blueberries into the batter, then pour the batter into the prepared baking pan. Top with the remaining berries. Bake in the preheated oven for 45 to 55 minutes, or until a knife comes out clean.

Cool on a wire rack for at least 30 minutes, then slice and enjoy!

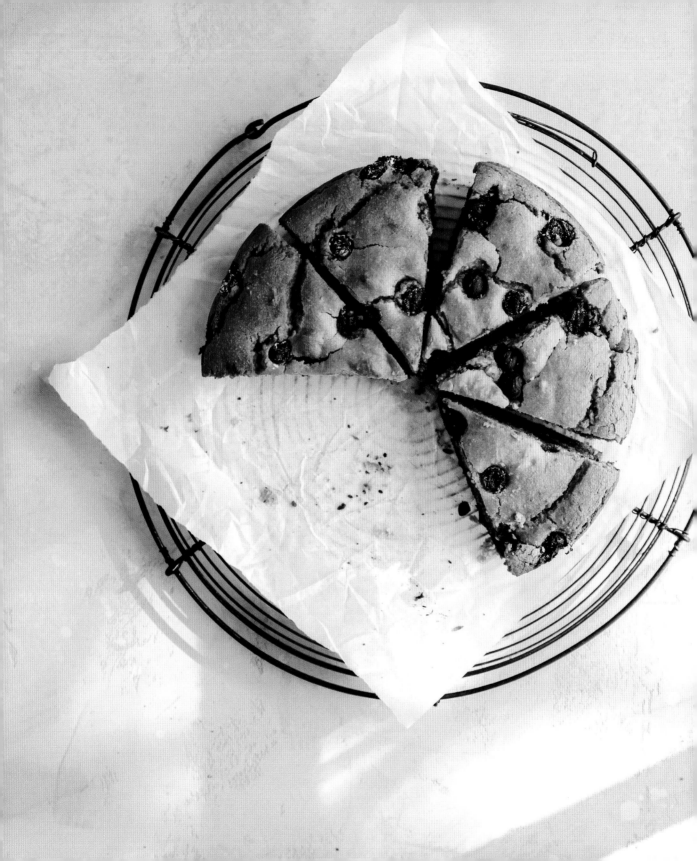

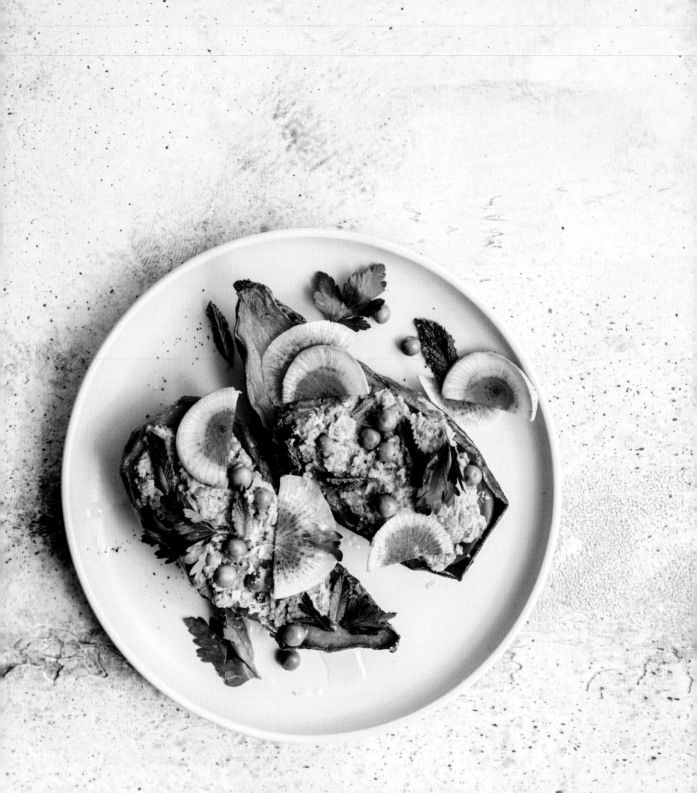

SWEET POTATO WEDGES WITH LEMONY CRUSHED PEAS

Smashed peas on toast was something I'd never seen until I moved to New York. I was skeptical that anything could come close to the quintessentially perfect avocado toast—hey, it's popular for a reason—but I was pleasantly surprised by how much I love this alternative topping. Here I've opted for the Paleo-friendly sweet potato wedge instead of toast, which I like to meal prep at the beginning of the week to enjoy with hummus, avocado or, of course, crushed peas.

Serves: 4

FOR THE SWEET POTATOES

2 large sweet potatoes

1 tbsp (15 ml) olive oil

FOR THE CRUSHED PEAS

2½ cups (362 g) green peas

½ cup (120 ml) water, plus more as needed

3 tbsp (45 ml) olive oil

Juice from ½ lemon

¼ tsp garlic powder

2 tbsp (7 g) finely chopped fresh parsley

2 tbsp (12 g) finely chopped fresh mint

FOR SERVING

Zest of 1 lemon

Maldon sea salt

Preheat the oven to 425°F (218°C). Line a baking sheet with parchment paper.

To make the sweet potatoes: Cut the sweet potatoes in half and drizzle with the oil. Place the sweet potatoes cut side down on the baking sheet and bake for 25 to 35 minutes, or until soft.

To make the crushed peas: Place the peas and water in a small saucepan. Bring the peas to a low boil for about 5 minutes. Drain the peas and rinse under cool water. Set about ¼ cup (36 g) of peas aside.

Add the rest of the peas to a food processor with the oil, lemon juice, garlic powder, parsley and mint. Pulse the pea mixture until smooth. Add 1 to 2 tablespoons (15 to 30 ml) of water if the mixture is too dry.

To serve: Stir in the reserved peas and then spread on the sweet potato wedges. Top with lemon zest and salt.

SAVORY KALE AND PROSCIUTTO CREPES

The first time I tried crepes I was eighteen years old running along the Canal Saint-Martin in Paris with three of my hostel roommates. It was the best and worst way to be introduced to crepes because they were so inexplicably perfect, but I've also never been able to experience anything quite on that level all these years later. While I can't claim to have mastered a recipe that perfectly resembles Parisian crepes, these are my go-to solution when the Paris nostalgia creeps in. Bonus: You can make these savory or sweet by swapping out the filling.

Serves: 4

FOR THE CREPES

3 eggs, room temperature

1 cup (120 ml) milk, room temperature

1 tbsp (15 ml) melted coconut oil

⅓ cup (43 g) cassava flour

¼ cup (24 g) almond flour

¼ cup (30 g) tapioca starch

¼ tsp sea salt

Coconut oil, for cooking

FOR THE FILLING

1 cup (100 g) shredded pecorino or cheese of choice (dairy-free, if needed)

8 slices of prosciutto

2 tbsp (30 ml) olive oil

2 cups (140 g) sliced baby bella mushrooms

2 cups (134 g) torn kale

FOR SERVING

Fresh herbs (I use chives and parsley.)

Maldon sea salt

To make the crepes: Whisk together the eggs and milk in a large bowl. Stir in the melted coconut oil, then add the cassava flour, almond flour, tapioca starch and salt. Whisk until the batter is smooth.

Grease a large skillet with coconut oil and place over medium heat. Pour about a ¼ cup (60 ml) of the crepe batter onto the pan and tilt it to create a thin, even circle.

Cook the crepe for about 1 minute, then flip it with a spatula and cook it on the other side for 1 minute. Repeat with the rest of the batter, greasing the pan with coconut oil as needed between crepes. This recipe makes eight crepes.

To make the filling: Place a scoop of cheese and a slice of prosciutto in a warm crepe and fold in half. Place the oil in a large skillet over medium heat along with the mushrooms. Sauté for 2 to 3 minutes to caramelize, then add the kale and continue to sauté for about 2 minutes, until wilted.

To serve: Serve the mushrooms and kale over the folded crepes. Top with fresh herbs and salt.

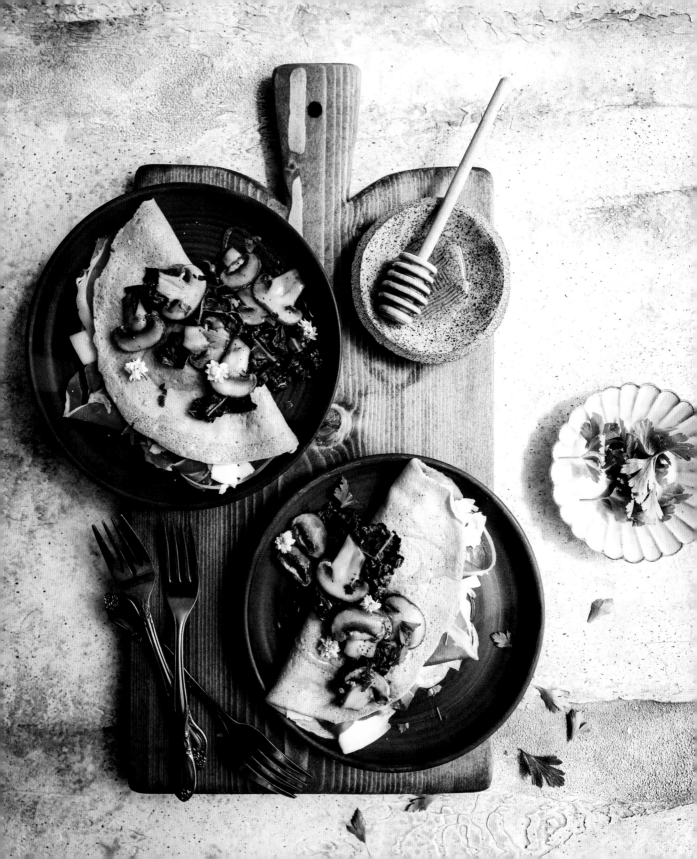

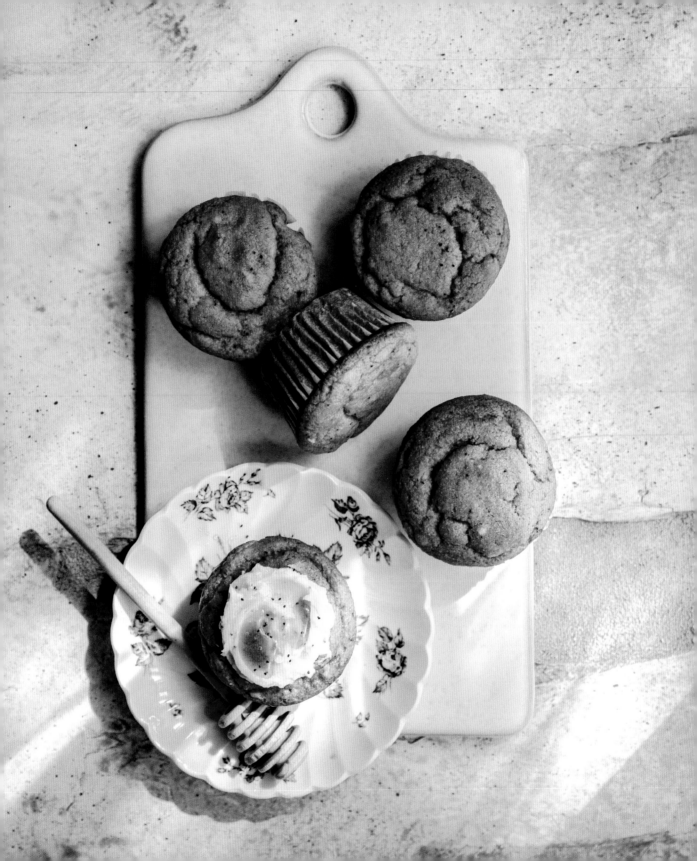

LEMON POPPY SEED MUFFINS

Nothing opens up tired eyes quite like a large cup of coffee and a lemon poppy seed muffin. What is more, there isn't a single time of year when a lemon poppy seed muffin seems out of place. They're the chocolate chip cookies of muffins: a staple owned by no season or holiday. After more than ten years of gluten-free baking experiments, I've arrived at a place where I nearly always bake with sweet potato purée and cassava flour combined, and these muffins are no exception. This unconventional ingredient combo makes a delightfully moist and sweet muffin that lets the lemon zest shine through.

Yield: 10 medium muffins

Juice of 1 lemon

⅓ cup (79 ml) coconut milk

2 large eggs

½ cup (127 g) cooked mashed Japanese sweet potato (skin removed)

¾ cup (150 g) coconut sugar or organic cane sugar

¼ cup (60 ml) olive oil

1 tsp vanilla extract

1 tsp baking soda

½ tsp cream of tartar

½ tsp sea salt

1 cup (130 g) cassava flour

¼ cup (30 g) tapioca starch

1 tbsp (9 g) poppy seeds

Preheat the oven to 350°F (177°C). Line a muffin tray with ten cupcake liners. Stir the lemon juice into the coconut milk and set aside.

Add the eggs, sweet potato, sugar, oil and vanilla to a blender. Blend for about 30 seconds, until smooth. Empty the mixture into a mixing bowl. Stir in the baking soda, cream of tartar and salt. Pour in the coconut milk mixture and stir to combine.

Add the cassava flour and tapioca starch to the bowl. Stir to combine. Fold the poppy seeds into the batter, then spoon the batter into the liners, leaving them about three-quarters of the way full. Bake in the oven for 22 to 25 minutes, or until a knife inserted into a muffin comes out clean. Cool on a wire rack for at least 30 minutes.

NOTE: Gluten-free muffins can be crumbly or soggy if enjoyed too quickly out of the oven. Let them cool on a wire rack completely. Store any leftovers in an airtight container for up to 4 days, or freeze for up to 3 months for a longer shelf life.

ZA'ATAR BREAKFAST SKILLET

Like most of my favorite foods, I discovered za'atar in New York City while dining out in SoHo on a business trip one winter. It was served with a hearty drizzle of olive oil over a side of unassuming vegetables that were waiting to blow my mind. One bite in and I was Googling what za'atar was, and promptly made my own take on the Lebanese spice blend once I was home. If you're anything like me, you also probably have everything on hand already! It's the perfect way to top off just about any vegetable dish, and it adds a new life to this quick and easy breakfast skillet.

Serves: 4

FOR THE ZA'ATAR

2 tbsp (18 g) sesame seeds

2 tbsp (5 g) dried thyme

2 tsp (3 g) ground sumac

1 tsp ground cumin

½ tsp sea salt

FOR THE SKILLET

2 tbsp (30 ml) olive oil

2 cloves garlic, minced

¼ cup (40 g) diced sweet onion

½ red bell pepper, diced

1 lb (454 g) merguez sausage or ground meat/sausage of choice

4 cups (268 g) spinach or kale

2 tbsp (6 g) za'atar

4 fried eggs

FOR SERVING

Toasted grain-free bread (optional)

To make the za'atar: In a small bowl, stir together the sesame seeds, thyme, sumac, cumin and salt. Store in a spice jar.

To make the skillet: Heat the oil in a large skillet over medium heat. Add the garlic, onion and bell pepper. Sauté for 2 to 3 minutes, or until tender.

Add the merguez sausage and sauté for 6 minutes, until no longer pink. Add the spinach and sauté for 4 to 5 minutes, until wilted. Sprinkle the za'atar over the skillet and stir to incorporate.

To serve: Divide the hash into four bowls and top each with a fried egg and za'atar. Serve with toasted bread, if desired.

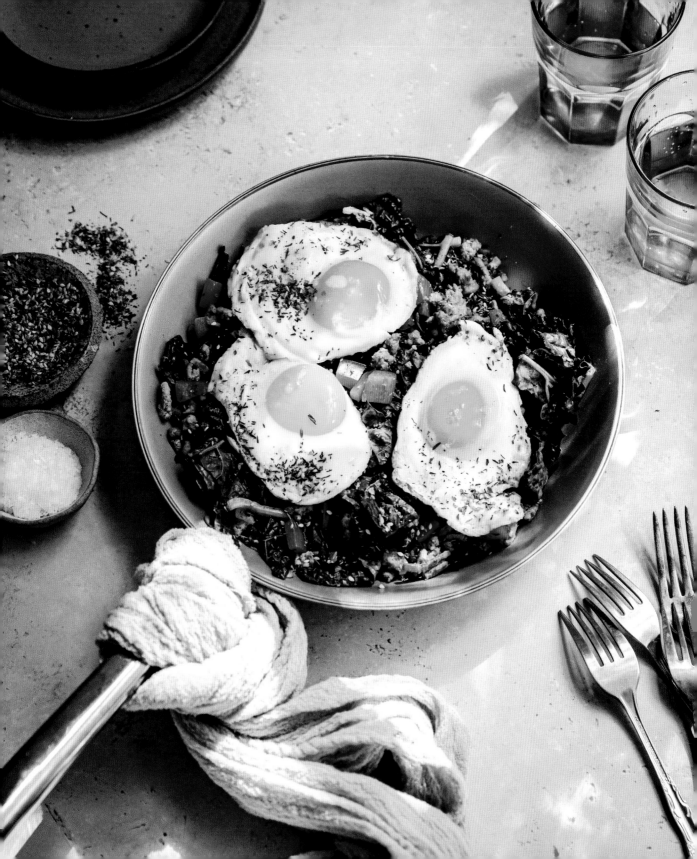

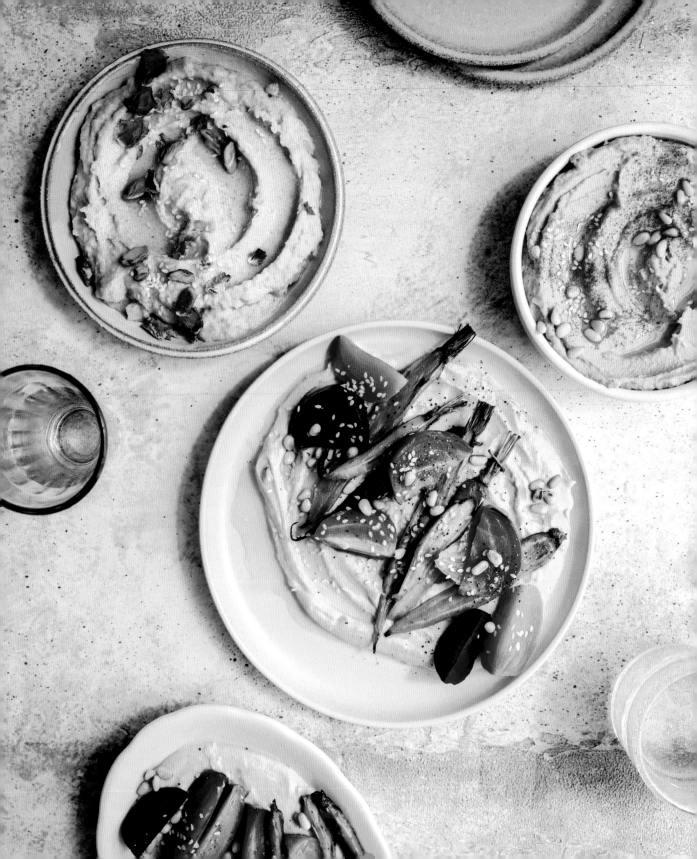

STAPLE DIPS AND SAUCES

I'm of the school of thought that says you can never have too many dips or sauces in your life. They can save an abysmally boring dish and turn it into a delight, and you can throw an excellent party if you fill the table with enough good Spicy Grapefruit Guacamole (page 133) and Spicy Sweet Potato Hummus (page 122) to share. They're also excellent comfort food, especially when you live in the gluten-free world.

Sometimes the best cooking isn't a grand gesture. Sometimes it is a bowl of perfectly blended hummus and a sweet potato chip. And sometimes that is exactly what you need.

PALEO HUMMUS WITH ROASTED BEETS AND CARROTS

One of my defining character traits is my unequivocal love of hummus. Hummus just *understands* me, and I'd like it to think I understand it equally in return. Hummus also understands roasted root vegetables, specifically beets and crispy carrots, though I have a feeling it would get along with whatever is in season at your local farmers' market. I like to serve my hummus with those roasted roots piled artistically on top. The result is as delicious and satisfying as it is beautiful.

Serves: 4

FOR THE BEETS AND CARROTS

4–5 small beets

6–8 small/medium carrots, peeled

2 tbsp (30 ml) olive oil

FOR THE HUMMUS

3 cups (300 g) cauliflower florets

⅓ cup (79 ml) tahini

3 tbsp (45 ml) olive oil

2 cloves garlic, minced

2 tbsp (30 ml) fresh lemon juice

½ tsp sea salt

FOR SERVING

2 tbsp (16 g) pine nuts

1 tbsp (9 g) sesame seeds

Olive oil, for drizzling

Preheat the oven to 400°F (204°C). Line a baking sheet with parchment paper.

To make the beets and carrots: Wrap the beets in a tight tinfoil packet and place them in the oven for 60 to 75 minutes, or until fork-tender. While the beets are cooking, toss the carrots on the baking sheet with oil to coat evenly and arrange them in a single layer. Place them in the oven when the beets have 25 minutes left, roasting until they are crispy and tender.

Slip the skins off the cooked beets and cut them into wedges, then toss them with the carrots. Set aside.

To make the hummus: Steam or roast the cauliflower florets, until softened. I steam mine for about 8 minutes. Add the steamed cauliflower, tahini, oil, garlic, lemon juice and salt to a food processor or high-speed blender. Blend until smooth.

To serve: Spread the hummus out on a platter and top with the roasted beets and carrots. Sprinkle with pine nuts, sesame seeds and an extra drizzle of olive oil.

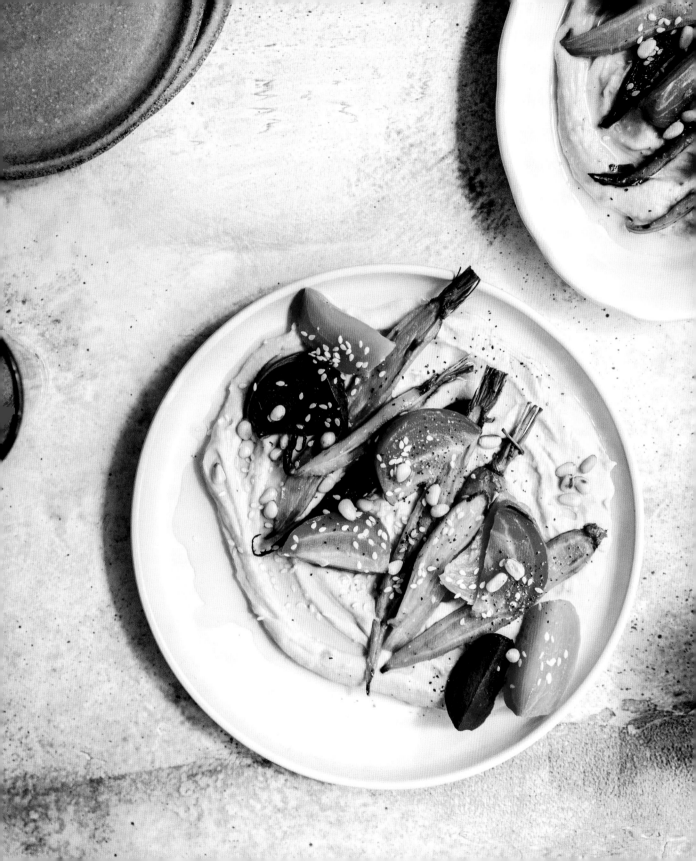

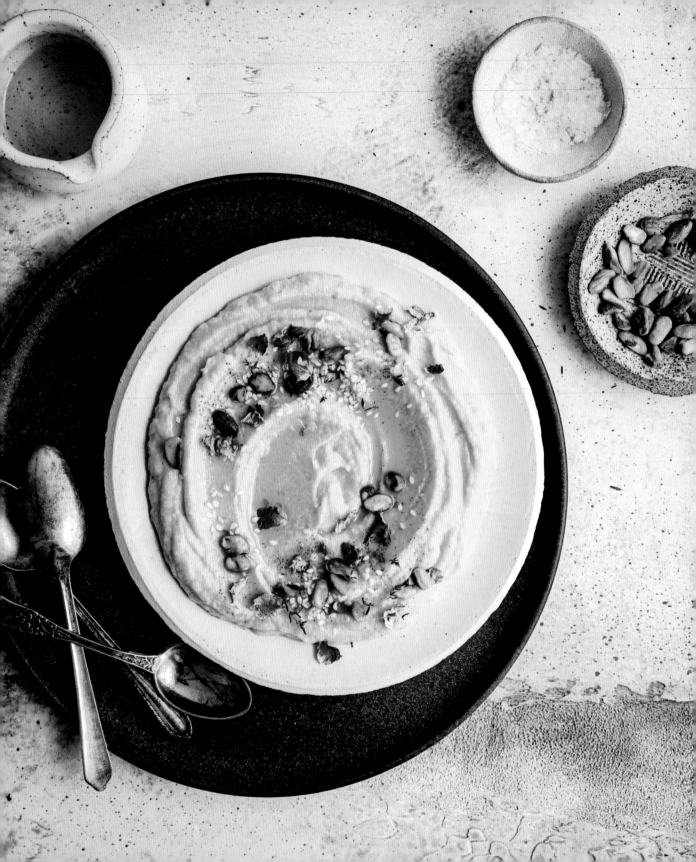

GOLDEN BEET DIP

My food photography and my recipes often inform each other, and both stem from an artistic sensibility that loves nuance and contrast. I brainstorm in a mix of flavors and colors, thinking about taste and about the layers that make a photo visually interesting. A beet dip sounds one-dimensional, but I love the mix of the sweet golden beets, creamy tahini and nutty pistachios. I also like to top this dip with edible rose petals for a colorful garnish when serving to guests. I make this on a weekly basis and consider it a small crisis if I open the fridge and find I've run out.

Serves: 4

FOR THE BEET DIP

4 medium golden beets (about 1 lb [454 g])

1 large shallot, peeled

2 tbsp (30 ml) olive oil

2 tbsp (30 ml) tahini

1 tbsp (15 ml) lemon juice

½ tsp paprika

½ tsp sea salt

FOR SERVING

2 tbsp (16 g) toasted pistachios

1 tbsp (9 g) sesame seeds

1 tbsp (3 g) edible rose petals (optional)

Preheat the oven to 400°F (204°C).

To make the beet dip: Wrap the beets and shallot in tinfoil and place on a baking sheet. Bake for 45 minutes, or until the beets are fork-tender. Slip the skins off the beets once they are cool enough to handle.

Add the beets, shallot, oil, tahini, lemon juice, paprika and salt to a food processor or high-speed blender. Blend until smooth.

To serve: Top with the toasted pistachios, sesame seeds and a sprinkle of rose petals (if using).

NOTE: I love golden beets for their color, but this works just as well with red beets!

SPICY SWEET POTATO HUMMUS

Here is what I know to be true: you do not need an occasion or a potluck of any kind to make yourself some delightful hummus. Don't wait for your neighbor to ask you to bring an app; make it when it's just you on a Tuesday. And since you're making hummus, make it with sweet potato and harissa—a delightful combination that you need more of in your life. Can you omit the harissa? Sure, this would still be a flavorful dip. But I find the sweet and smoky harissa to be deal-making-and-breaking perfection that I would only omit if all of Manhattan was out of stock.

Serves: 4 to 6

FOR THE HUMMUS

3 cups (300 g) cauliflower florets

Flesh of 1 large cooked sweet potato

1 heaping tbsp (9 g) harissa paste

⅓ cup (80 ml) tahini

2 tbsp (30 ml) olive oil

½ tsp paprika, plus more for topping

2 cloves garlic, minced

¼ tsp sea salt

FOR SERVING

2 tbsp (16 g) toasted pine nuts

1 tbsp (9 g) sesame seeds

To make the hummus: Steam or cook the cauliflower florets, until softened. I steam mine for about 10 minutes.

Add the cauliflower, sweet potato, harissa, tahini, oil, paprika, garlic and salt to a food processor or high-speed blender. Blend until smooth.

To serve: Top with pine nuts, sesame seeds and an extra sprinkle of paprika.

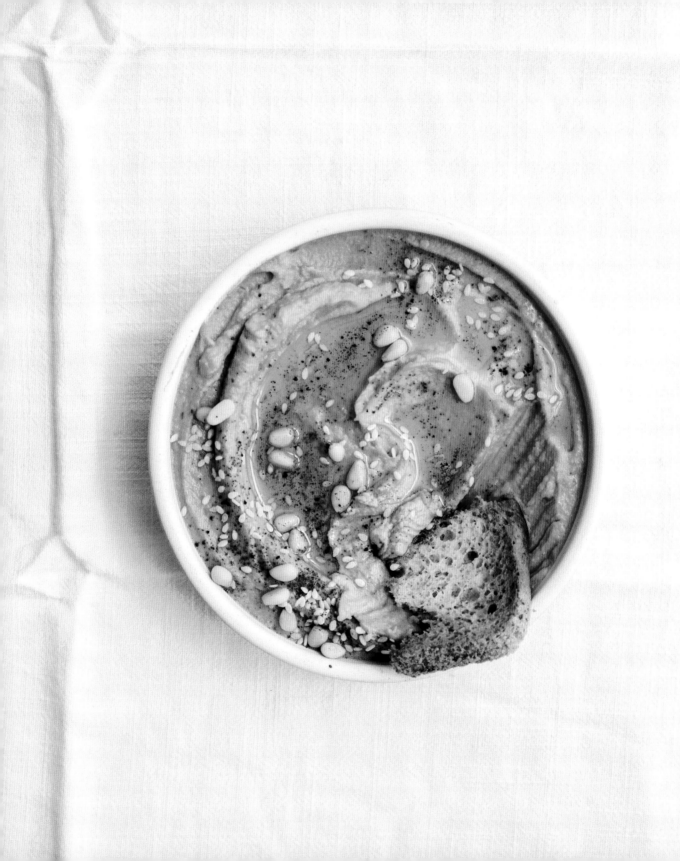

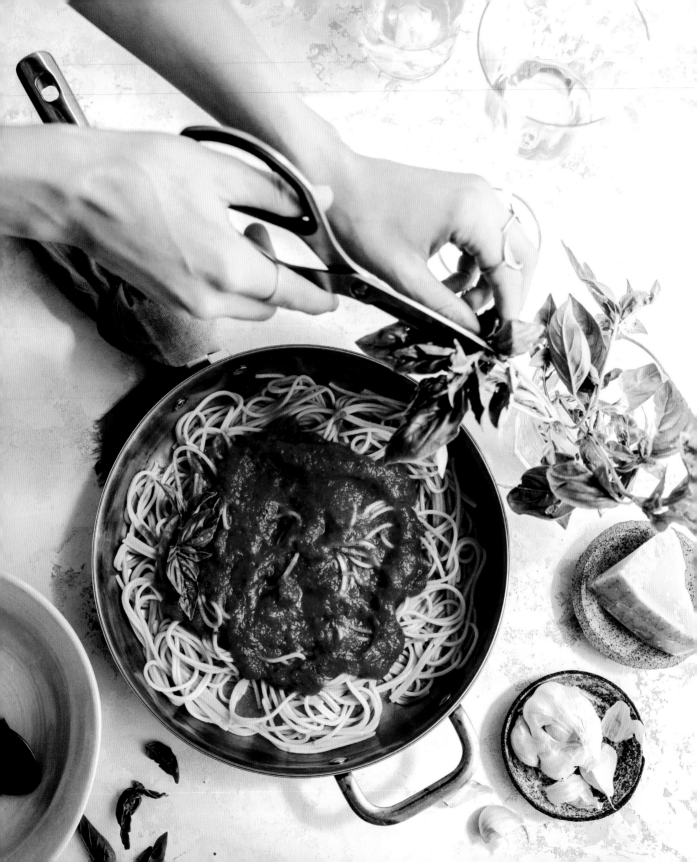

APARTMENT ARRABBIATA

I was not raised around cooking with one exception: *the* red sauce. I remember sitting on the kitchen island holding the off-white spatula and begging my mom to let me pour in all of the ingredients that went into this labor of love that would simmer on the stovetop all afternoon, filling the house with the smell of herbs and garlic. I've long forgotten the specific recipe, though I'm sure it's scribbled on a yellowed index card somewhere in a drawer in my parent's home. I've paid tribute to this memory by making what I nicknamed my "Apartment Arrabbiata," a red sauce that is easy to make when you live in an NYC walkup that has zero counter space, or when you simply don't have the patience for a complicated sauce.

Serves: 8

3 tbsp (45 ml) olive oil

4 cloves garlic, minced

2 (28-oz [793-g]) cans San Marzano tomatoes with liquid

½ cup (120 ml) dry white wine

1 tsp salt

1 tsp red pepper flakes

Place the oil in a large pot over medium heat. Add the garlic to the pot and sauté for 2 to 3 minutes. Add the tomatoes, wine, salt and red pepper flakes.

Simmer the sauce for 20 minutes, stirring occasionally and breaking up the tomatoes. Serve over pasta or use the sauce in your recipe of choice.

NOTE: You can keep this sauce covered in the fridge for up to 1 week, or freeze it for up to 3 months.

COMPOTE THREE WAYS

There is always a compote on hand in my refrigerator—always. It's cheap, easy and requires minimal ingredients, so we get along great. Each week I browse the farmers' market for a fun new fruit to take home and cook down for the week, but I always come back to one of these three combos. Though blueberry is definitely my favorite, if you're asking.

Yield: about 1 cup (about 380 g)

FOR THE BLUEBERRY COMPOTE

2½ cups (444 g) blueberries

¼ cup (60 ml) water

1 tbsp (15 ml) lemon juice

FOR THE CINNAMON PEAR COMPOTE

3 pears, peeled, cored and chopped

2 tbsp (30 ml) water

1 tbsp (15 ml) maple syrup

½ tsp ground cinnamon

¼ tsp ground nutmeg

¼ tsp sea salt

FOR THE PEACH BASIL COMPOTE

4 peaches, peeled and sliced with pits removed

¼ cup (60 ml) water

¼ tsp sea salt

2 tbsp (6 g) chopped fresh basil

To make the compote: Combine all the ingredients for your desired compote in a saucepan over medium heat. If you are making the peach basil compote, combine all of the ingredients but the basil.

Bring to a boil, then reduce the heat to a low simmer. Stir and simmer for 5 to 10 minutes, or until the compote is reduced and thickened.

Remove the compote from the heat and allow it to cool. For the peach compote, stir in the basil after cooking. Serve or store covered in the fridge for up to 6 days.

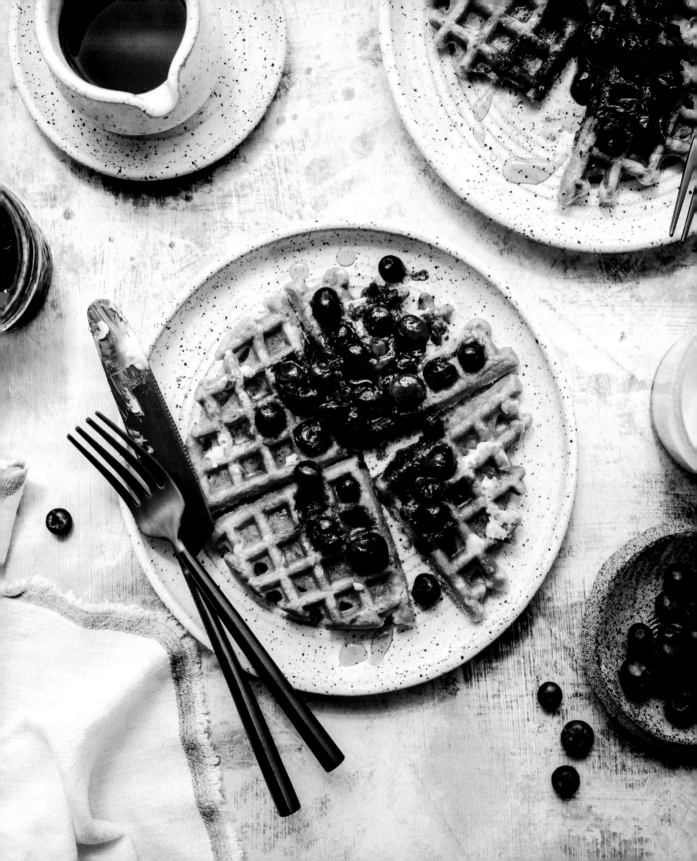

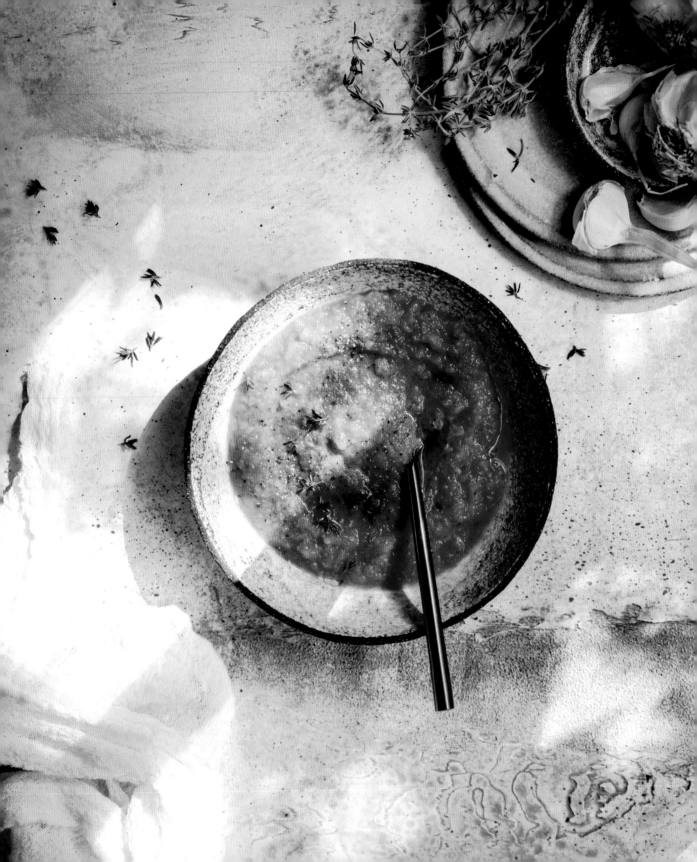

NUT-FREE ROMESCO

Look, you should always have a dip on hand in the fridge ready to go. This is a fact of life. Dips are the emergency kit for meals, the go-to problem solver when things are bland and boring. But I know that dips can get tricky when you are avoiding nuts and seed oils— because as much as we all love guac, it's not exactly a sustainable fridge staple. Traditional romesco is made with nuts, but this is my nut-free version for those of us that need it. Keep this in your fridge for a few days and use it to liven up your meals.

Serves: 4

FOR THE ROMESCO

2 large red bell peppers, quartered and de-seeded

½ sweet onion, chopped

2 cloves garlic

3 tbsp (45 ml) olive oil

1 tbsp (15 ml) lemon juice

1 tbsp (5 g) nutritional yeast

½ tsp sea salt

½ tsp paprika

FOR SERVING (OPTIONAL)

Citrus Roasted Chicken Thighs with Artichokes (page 32)

Vegetables

Crackers

To make the romesco: Preheat the oven to 425°F (218°C) and line a baking sheet with parchment paper. Toss the bell peppers, onion and garlic with the oil. Spread the vegetables evenly on the baking sheet and place it in the oven for 25 minutes, until tender and beginning to char, tossing halfway through.

Place the roasted vegetables in a food processor with the lemon juice, nutritional yeast, salt and paprika. Purée until smooth, scraping down the sides as needed.

To serve: Plate the romesco and top with chicken thighs, or serve as a dip alongside vegetables or crackers. You can also keep your romesco in an airtight jar in the fridge for up to 4 days.

PESTO THREE WAYS

Pesto may well be my love language. It's an effective one, too. Pesto is the mellow, personable, non-abrasive friend that you can bring to any party and know that they'll fit right in. There's hardly a dish out there that doesn't go great with a side of pesto, no matter what time of day it is. And just to prove my point, you can make pesto using pretty much any combination of greens, nuts and seeds you have on hand. Here are three of my favorite ways.

Yield: 1 cup (260 g)

FOR THE CASHEW BASIL PESTO

2 cups (48 g) fresh basil

1 cup (20 g) arugula

⅓ cup (49 g) cashews

3 tbsp (45 ml) olive oil

½ tsp sea salt, plus more to taste

1 clove garlic

2 tbsp (30 ml) fresh lemon juice

2 tbsp (10 g) nutritional yeast

FOR THE KALE PARMESAN PESTO

2 cups (134 g) curly kale

⅓ cup (80 ml) olive oil

¼ cup (35 g) pine nuts

2 tbsp (30 ml) lemon juice

¼ cup (25 g) Parmesan or 2 tbsp (10 g) nutritional yeast

½ tsp sea salt, plus more to taste

FOR THE BROCCOLI ALMOND PESTO

1 cup (91 g) chopped broccoli florets

2 tbsp (19 g) almonds

½ cup (30 g) fresh parsley

2 tbsp (10 g) nutritional yeast

2 tbsp (30 ml) lemon juice

⅓ cup (80 ml) olive oil

2 cloves garlic

½ tsp sea salt, plus more to taste

To make the pesto: Place all of the ingredients for the desired pesto in a food processor or blender. Blend for 2 minutes, or until smooth. Add salt to taste, if needed.

Keep leftover pesto in an airtight container in the fridge for up to 5 days.

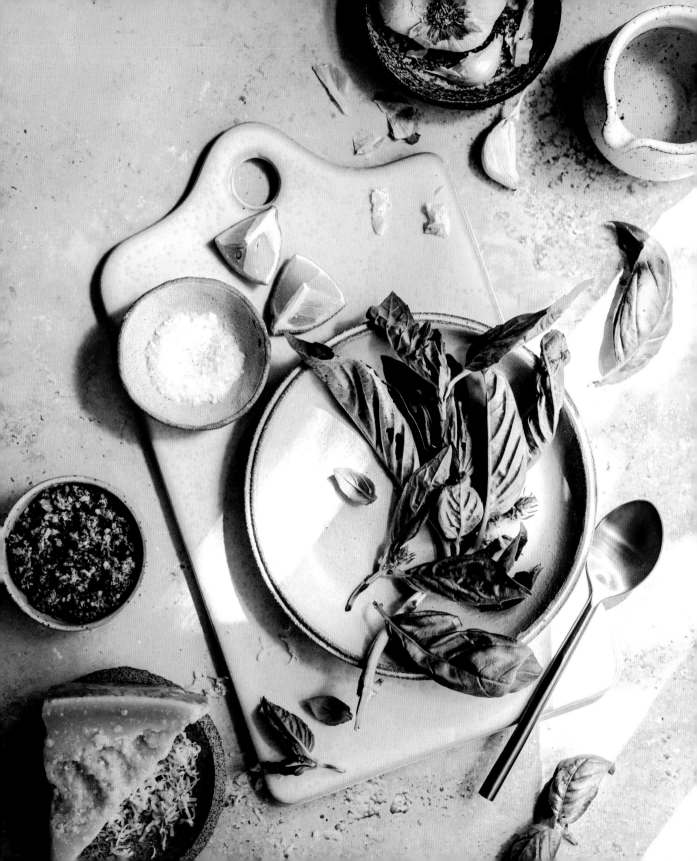

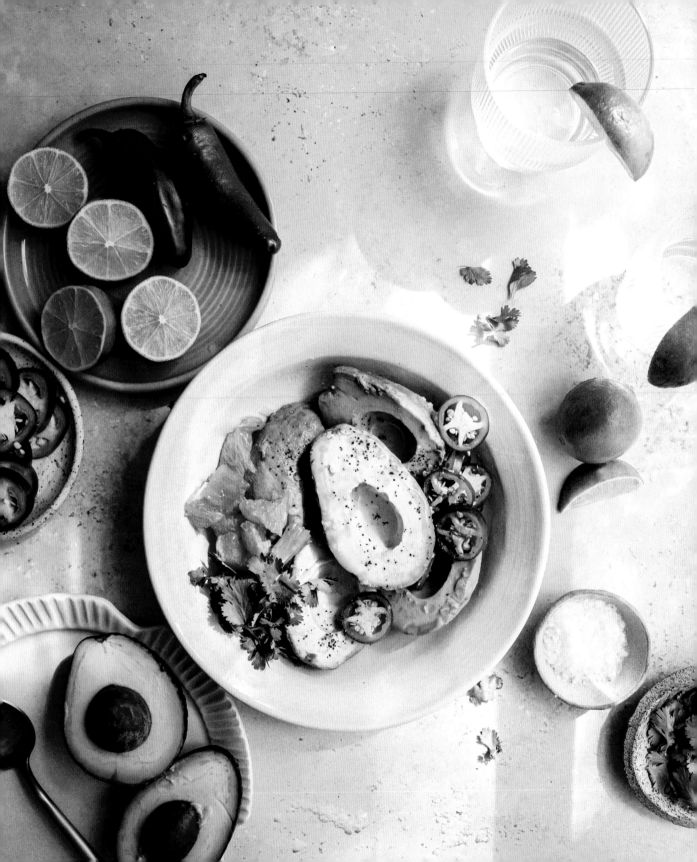

SPICY GRAPEFRUIT GUACAMOLE

I'm going to break the cookbook fourth wall for a minute here and acknowledge that I'm writing this on a New York City sidewalk during the COVID-19 pandemic. It's been a year since the day I last had friends over for a girls' night where we sat around and ate a large bowl of this grapefruit guacamole. I remember the patio doors flung open and the twinkle lights plugged in, and I remember scraping every last bit of guac up with my cucumber slice and laughing until I couldn't breathe. There are good things that come from isolation, this book being one of them. But there are tastes that are only realized when a meal is enjoyed across from the smiles of others. I can't wait for nights like that again.

Serves: 6

3 large ripe avocados, halved, seeded and peeled

Juice of 1 lime

1 clove garlic, minced

1 grapefruit, sliced, removed from membrane and cut into chunks, plus more for garnish

¼ cup (15 g) finely chopped fresh cilantro

½ tsp sea salt

¼ tsp black pepper

1 small jalapeño, seeded and chopped, plus more for garnish

Place the avocados and lime juice in a medium-sized bowl and mash well with a fork. Add the garlic, grapefruit chunks, cilantro, salt and pepper. Stir to combine. Gently fold in the jalapeño.

Garnish with grapefruit or jalapeño, if desired.

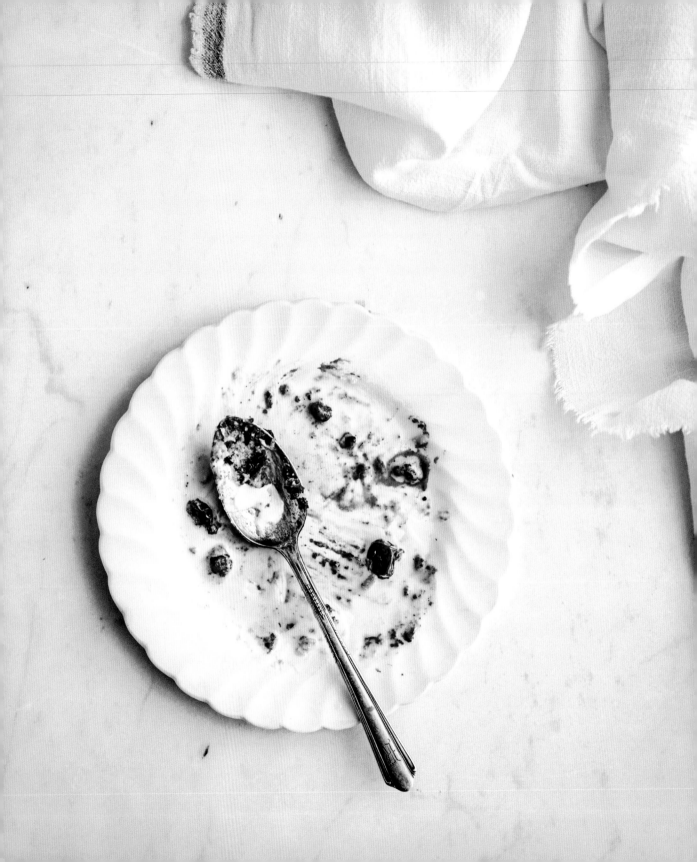

INDULGENCES AND DESSERTS

Full disclosure: I am not a dessert person. I try hard to be, but it's just not something I'm invested in. Maybe it's because I don't love baking, so I'd much rather put my energy into making a meal and then call it a day. I DO love puppies and sunshine, so I promise I'm not an entirely dark, sinister soul.

What got me psyched to write this chapter was the idea of contrast and flavors that taste like holidays and birthdays. They say that smell is the strongest memory, and there is something nostalgic and comforting about the smell of Tahini Zucchini Bread (page 144) or Peach Cobbler (page 147) in the oven that brings me back to simpler times. Hopefully these recipes bring back sweet memories for you, too.

BERRY CRISP WITH MAPLE SAUCE

Crisps, cobblers and crumbles are my favorite desserts. They remind me of seemingly endless summer days where the sun lingers just a bit longer over patio dinners in the New England summer air. I usually make blueberry-focused crisps that remind me of Maine blueberries, but ultimately this crisp can be made with whatever berry—or berries—you have on hand!

Serves: 6 to 8

FOR THE MAPLE SAUCE

2 tbsp (30 ml) tahini, almond butter or nut butter of choice

3 tbsp (45 ml) maple syrup

Pinch of salt

FOR THE FILLING

6 cups (888 g) berries of choice (I use half blueberries and half blackberries.)

1 tbsp (15 ml) lemon juice

1 tsp vanilla extract

1 tbsp (7 g) tapioca starch

FOR THE TOPPING

⅔ cup (86 g) cassava flour

⅓ cup (65 g) coconut sugar or organic cane sugar

½ cup (54 g) slivered almonds

½ tsp sea salt

¼ cup plus 1 tbsp (69 g) coconut oil

FOR SERVING

Coconut milk ice cream

To make the maple sauce: Whisk together the tahini, maple syrup and salt in a small bowl until smooth. Set aside.

Preheat the oven to 375°F (190°C). Grease an 8- or 9-inch (20- or 23-cm) baking dish with coconut oil.

To make the filling: In a large bowl, mix the berries, lemon juice, vanilla and tapioca starch. Pour the berries into the prepared dish.

To make the topping: In a separate bowl, stir together the cassava flour, coconut sugar, almonds and salt. Add the coconut oil and use a fork to cut it into the flour mixture until well mixed and crumbly. Sprinkle the flour mixture evenly over the berries.

Place the crisp in the oven and bake for 30 minutes, or until the fruit is bubbly and the top is golden.

To serve: Allow the crisp to cool for 10 minutes. Serve with coconut milk ice cream and the maple sauce.

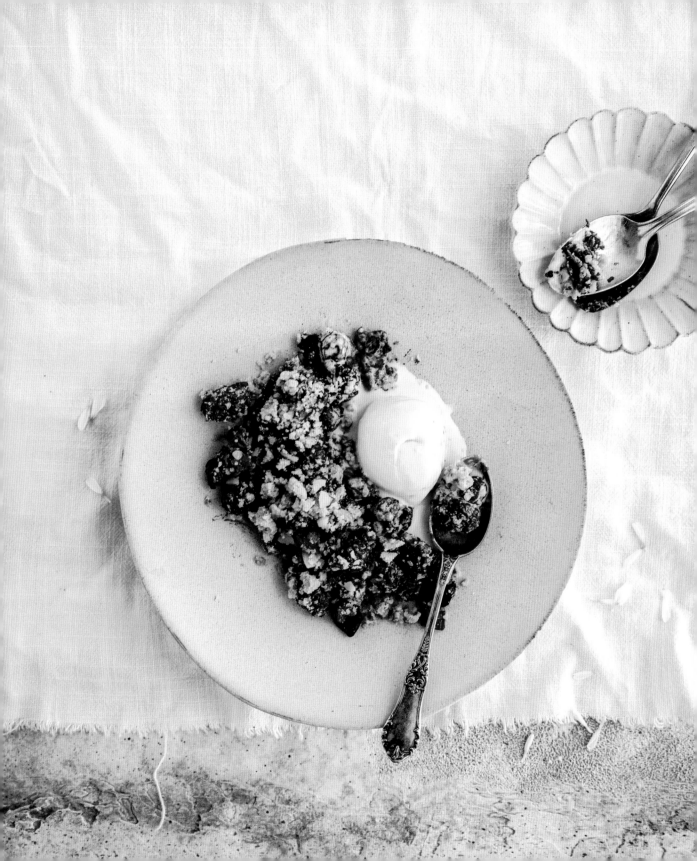

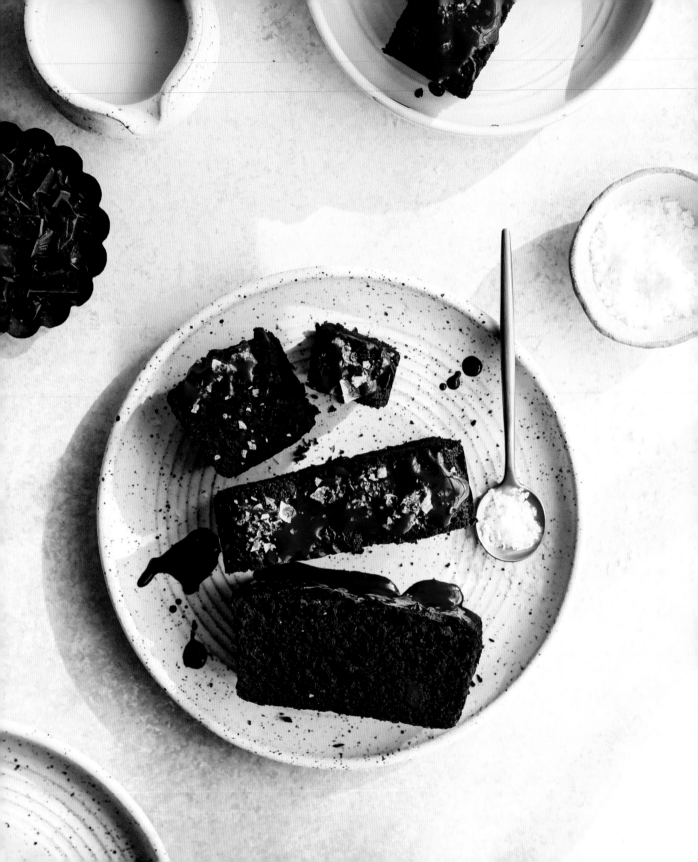

EXTRA THICK AND FUDGY SWEET POTATO BROWNIES

There is a delightful nostalgia in brownies that I'll never get over. They remind me of backyard summers and lemonade stands with friends when everything was funny. Someone's mom always brought out a Pyrex pan of brownies that disappeared too fast. These are a bit more like flourless cake with a flakey, crackly brownie top—more evolved brownies, if you will. The sweet potato keeps them rich and moist, and a generous amount of melted chocolate swirled into the batter makes them oh-so decadent. I bake mine in a loaf pan, which makes them extra thick and fudgy and is so worth the extra baking time.

Serves: 6 to 12

½ cup (44 g) unsweetened cocoa powder

½ cup (65 g) cassava flour

¼ tsp sea salt

¼ tsp baking soda

1 large egg, room temperature

¾ cup (150 g) coconut sugar or organic cane sugar

1 large cooked mashed sweet potato (I peel mine and steam until soft; about 1 cup [255 g].)

1½ cups (252 g) dairy-free chocolate chips, divided

⅓ cup (80 ml) melted coconut oil

Maldon sea salt, for topping

Preheat the oven to 350°F (176°C). Line a 9 x 5–inch (23 x 13–cm) loaf pan with parchment paper.

In a small bowl, whisk together the cocoa powder, cassava flour, salt and baking soda. Set aside.

In a medium bowl, use a mixer to beat the egg and sugar together for 2 minutes. Add the sweet potato and beat again for 1 to 2 minutes, or until the sweet potato is well combined and no longer "stringy." If you don't have a mixer, you can also achieve this in a blender.

Place 1 cup (168 g) of the chocolate chips and the coconut oil in a microwave-safe bowl and microwave in 20-second intervals, stirring in between, until melted.

Stir the chocolate mixture into the sweet potato batter until smooth. Add the cocoa powder mixture and mix until well combined. Fold in ¼ cup (42 g) of the remaining chocolate chips.

Pour the batter into the prepared pan and bake for 45 to 50 minutes, or until a knife comes out clean. Cool for 20 minutes in the pan, then transfer the brownies to a wire rack to cool for 20 minutes. Melt the remaining chocolate chips and drizzle on top. Finish with flakey salt and enjoy!

NOTES: For an extra special treat, slice the loaf into five to six thick slices. Or slice it in half lengthwise and then into five to six slices to serve a larger crowd. Part of the key to the crackly brownie top is to really beat your sugar into your egg so the sugar begins to dissolve. This makes a huge difference!

ROASTED GRAPEFRUIT WITH BRITTLE

Most of my cooking is based on elevating the basic magic of fresh ingredients. It's a fancy way of saying "I'm kind of lazy," but I digress. I love a dessert recipe based on cooked fruit with a hint of sugar to help caramelize it and a crunchy contrasting texture. No complicated mixing, folding or frosting. Here I've followed my basic magic/laziness formula to make a caramelized grapefruit topped off with an easy brittle. Pair it with some whipped cream for the perfect final touch. Or don't. It's all great either way.

Serves: 6

FOR THE BRITTLE

1 cup (143 g) roughly chopped almonds

2 cups (258 g) cashew pieces

¼ cup (34 g) sunflower seeds

1 tbsp (9 g) sesame seeds

¼ tsp sea salt

⅓ cup (80 ml) honey

1 tbsp (15 ml) melted coconut oil

FOR THE GRAPEFRUIT

3 grapefruit, sliced in half

¼ cup (50 g) coconut sugar

½ tsp (3 g) cinnamon

FOR SERVING

Coconut whipped cream

Preheat the oven to 350°F (177°C). Line a baking sheet with parchment paper.

To make the brittle: Stir together the almonds, cashews, sunflower seeds, sesame seeds and salt in a large mixing bowl. Add the honey and coconut oil. Stir to combine, then pour onto the baking sheet and press into a rectangle. Bake for 15 to 20 minutes, until golden. Set the pan aside to cool for 15 minutes, then break the brittle into pieces.

To make the grapefruit: Place the oven rack about 4 to 6 inches (10 to 15 cm) below the broiler and preheat the broiler. Place the grapefruit cut side up on a baking sheet, then coat it with sugar and cinnamon. Broil the grapefruit for 3 to 4 minutes, until bubbly and caramelized.

To serve: Serve the broiled grapefruit with whipped cream and brittle.

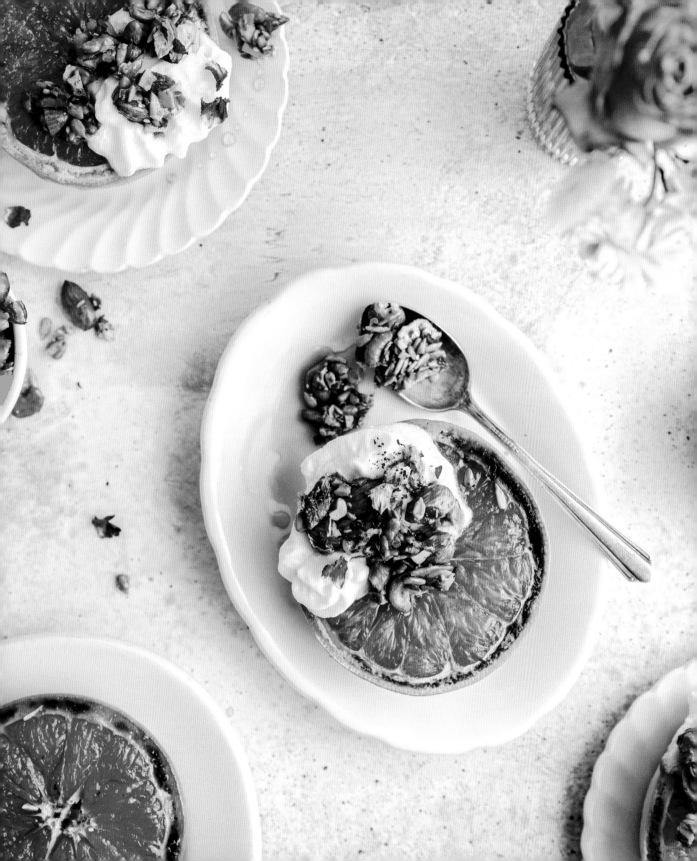

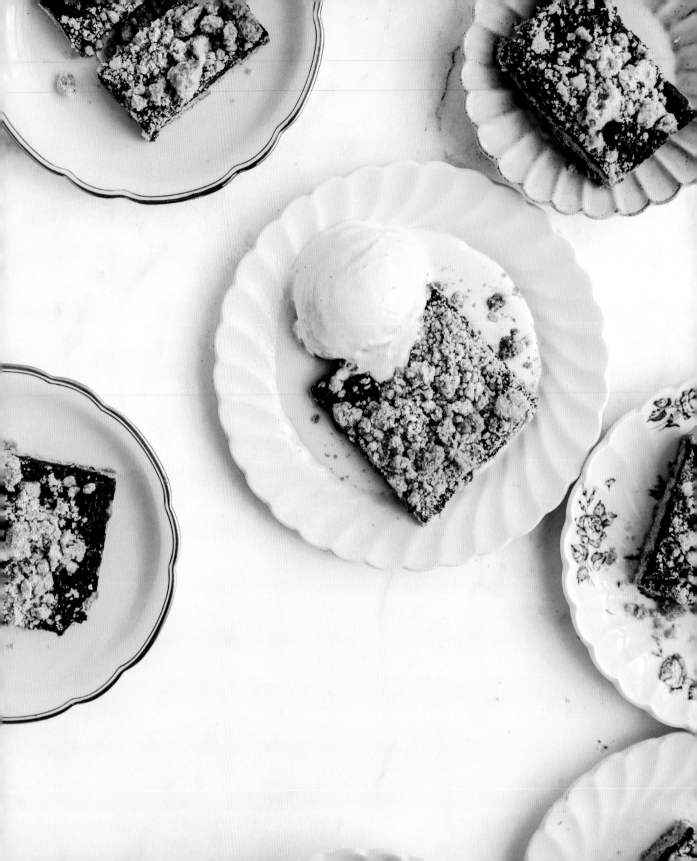

BLACKBERRY CRUMB BARS

Whenever I see pie my gut reaction is probably a bit different from everyone else's. I immediately think, "That crust looks like *work*." Maybe it's because I didn't grow up making much pie, but I've always been more drawn toward what I think of as "lazy pie," a.k.a. an easy shortbread bar with some cooked fruit and an easy crumble. I change the fruit out depending on the season, but blackberry is a current favorite that I've been using on repeat.

Serves: 12

FOR THE FILLING

1 lb (454 g) fresh blackberries

3 tbsp (38 g) coconut sugar or organic cane sugar

2 tbsp (30 ml) water

1 tbsp (15 ml) lemon juice

1 tbsp (7 g) tapioca starch

FOR THE CRUST

1½ cups (195 g) cassava flour

1 tbsp (7 g) coconut flour

½ tsp baking soda

¼ tsp sea salt

¼ cup (50 g) coconut sugar or organic cane sugar

½ cup (110 g) coconut oil, softened

1 egg

2–4 tbsp (30–60 ml) cold water

To make the filling: Place the blackberries in a saucepan over medium heat with the sugar, water and lemon juice. Cook for 7 to 8 minutes, stirring every few minutes and mashing with a spatula, until the blackberries are broken down and thickened. Remove from the heat and stir in the tapioca starch. Set aside.

Preheat the oven to 350°F (177°C). Line an 8 x 8–inch (20 x 20–cm) baking pan with parchment paper.

To make the crust: In a large bowl, whisk together the cassava flour, coconut flour, baking soda, salt and coconut sugar. Add the softened coconut oil and combine with a fork, until crumbly and well mixed. Stir in the egg and water until well combined. The batter will be crumbly, but it will hold together when pressed.

Set aside ⅓ cup (80 g) of the mixture for the crumble and press the rest of the dough into the bottom of the pan. Bake for 10 minutes. Top the prebaked crust with the blackberry mixture and sprinkle the reserved crumble evenly over the filling. Bake for 18 to 22 minutes, or until lightly browned.

Allow the bars to cool for at least 15 minutes. Remove from pan, slice and enjoy! Store any leftovers in the fridge for up to 5 days.

TAHINI ZUCCHINI BREAD

Once you go tahini, you never go back. So obviously tahini had to make its way into the desserts chapter, along with a cameo appearance by my beloved zucchini. What can I say? I'm loyal to a fault. The nutty richness of the tahini pairs perfectly with the sweet chocolate chunks, while the zucchini keeps this loaf perfectly moist. It's a satisfying flavor and texture composition that hits all the right notes.

Yield: 10 slices

1 tsp apple cider vinegar

¼ cup (60 ml) canned coconut milk

2 eggs, whisked

⅓ cup (80 ml) maple syrup

⅓ cup (66 g) coconut sugar or organic cane sugar

½ cup (120 ml) tahini

2 tbsp (30 ml) olive oil

1 tsp vanilla extract

1 tsp baking soda

½ tsp cream of tartar

¼ tsp sea salt

1 cup plus 2 tbsp (146 g) cassava flour

¼ cup (30 g) tapioca starch

1 medium zucchini, shredded

1 chocolate bar, chopped (1.8 oz or similar)

2 tbsp (18 g) sesame seeds

Preheat the oven to 350°F (177°C). Line a 9 x 5–inch (23 x 13–cm) loaf pan with parchment paper.

Stir the vinegar into the coconut milk and set aside. In a large bowl, whisk together the eggs, maple syrup and sugar until well combined. Add the tahini, oil and vanilla, and whisk again to incorporate.

Stir in the baking soda, cream of tartar and salt. Pour the coconut milk mixture over the top and stir to combine. Add the cassava flour and tapioca starch to the batter and mix.

Gently fold in the zucchini and chocolate, then pour the batter into the prepared pan.

Sprinkle the sesame seeds over the top of the batter. Bake for 45 to 50 minutes, or until a toothpick inserted into the center of the loaf comes out clean.

Let the loaf cool for 10 minutes, then remove it from the pan and cool on a wire rack for 1 hour.

NOTE: This bread needs to be cooled quite well before slicing or it'll seem too mushy. Leftovers will keep up for to 5 days in an airtight container.

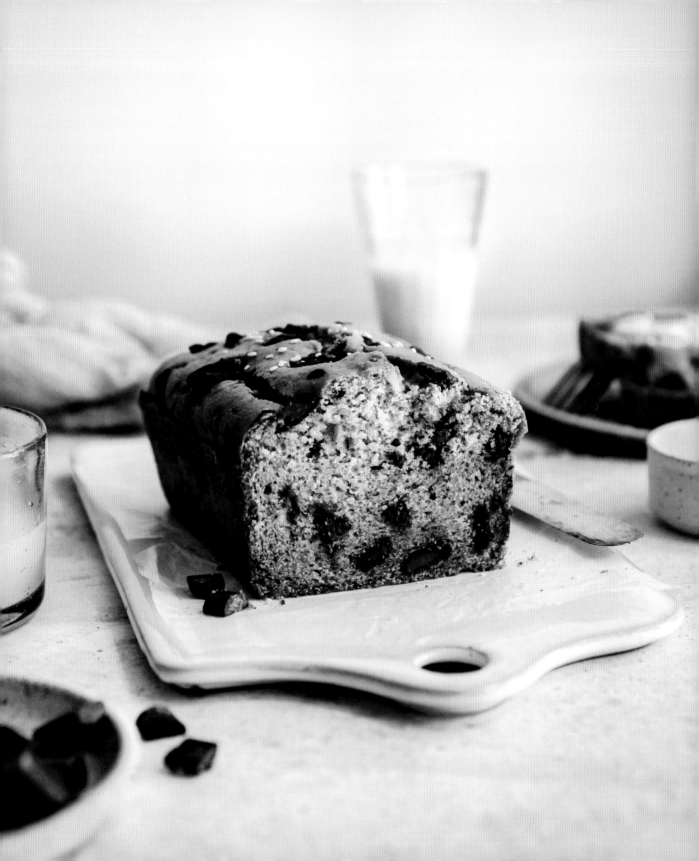

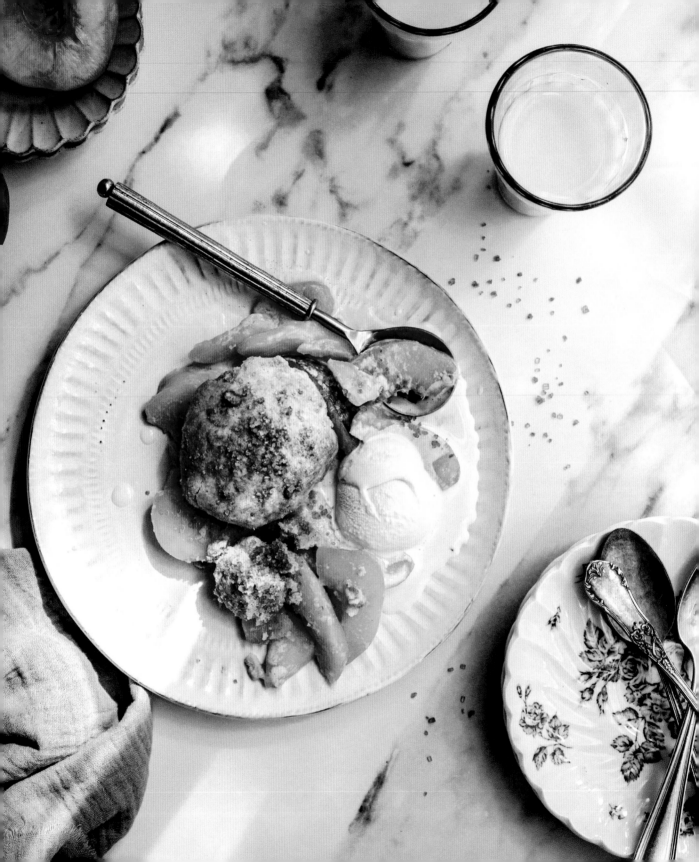

PEACH COBBLER

Peaches taste the way summer feels, and if you've ever had a perfectly ripe peach you know exactly what I'm talking about. Long shadows, dewy grass, bright afternoons, carefree beach days. Peaches encapsulate it all with resplendent flair. I'm ashamed to admit that I haven't given peaches enough appreciation in my life, but I assure you I'm working hard to make up for this transgression now. Case in point: I'm very protective of my cobbler recipe and only use it with fruit that I truly believe in, much in the way that Tarantino casts his movies. It takes a real talented soul to play the part. All of this to say, this recipe is a carefully written dessert production. You'll just swoon. It's too good.

Serves: 6

FOR THE FILLING

8 ripe peaches, pitted and sliced

2 tbsp (30 g) coconut sugar or organic cane sugar

1 tbsp (7 g) tapioca starch

Juice of ½ lemon

FOR THE COBBLER

1 tbsp (15 ml) fresh lemon juice

⅓ cup (80 ml) canned coconut milk

1¼ cups (163 g) cassava flour

⅓ cup (40 g) tapioca starch

¼ cup (50 g) coconut sugar or organic cane sugar

1 tsp baking soda

½ tsp cream of tartar

¼ tsp sea salt

½ cup (110 g) coconut oil

2 tbsp (26 g) coarse sanding sugar, for topping (Use coconut sugar for strict-Paleo.)

FOR SERVING

Coconut ice cream

Preheat the oven to 350°F (177°C). Grease a 9-inch (23-cm) baking dish with coconut oil.

To make the filling: Stir together the peaches, sugar, tapioca starch and lemon juice in a large bowl. When coated, add the fruit to the prepared dish.

To make the cobbler: Stir the lemon juice into the coconut milk. Set aside.

Whisk the cassava flour, tapioca starch, coconut sugar, baking soda, cream of tartar and salt in a large bowl.

Add the coconut oil to the bowl and cut it into the flour mixture with a fork until crumbly. Add the coconut milk mixture and stir until a thick dough forms.

Form six or seven biscuit-shaped balls and place them on top of the peaches to form a crust layer. Sprinkle the sanding sugar over the top of the biscuits.

Bake for 30 to 35 minutes, until the fruit is bubbly and the biscuits are golden.

To serve: Remove the cobbler from the oven and allow it to sit for 15 minutes to thicken. Serve warm with coconut ice cream!

ACKNOWLEDGMENTS

Mom and Dad, thanks for letting me dream without boundaries from the very beginning and tolerating a lifetime of my independence. Dad, you showed me what it is to work quietly and hard without an expectation of immediate success. Mom, you are living proof that art is valuable for both the audience and the artist. Thank you for letting me grow up in your museum.

Trent and Si, I'm not sure if I've told you, and it's a shame you'll never read this book, but you are my favorite people, and I'm so proud that I get to be your sister.

V, I am me because I grew up with you chasing creativity by my side.

Emily, you are the epitome of what it is to be a generous collaborator and editor. Thank you for seeing something in me when I was too afraid to send a pitch and for graciously and thoughtfully answering every last email.

Material Kitchen, thank you for noticing me when my pictures were still blurry and oversaturated and for giving me tools that make me actually want to cook.

New York City, maybe it's odd to thank a place full of people I've never met, but I couldn't imagine writing this book anywhere else. I never felt fully "me" until you became my home.

To all of the growers at Union Square Greenmarket, thank you endlessly for your kind eyes that have greeted me on all of the early mornings when I went looking for ingredients, and for answering my questions about herbs and beets.

To Hudson, you and your fluffy tail are my favorite coworkers. Thanks for keeping me company and keeping me smiling, and for leaving shoot food alone during work hours.

To all of the brands and restaurants who have let me photograph your products and dishes through my lens. There are too many of you to name here, but you've helped me live my dream and given me the practice to get to the point of writing this book. Thank you for demanding my best and helping me grow.

And to my readers for all of these years. You blow me away every day with your thoughtful questions and curious minds. Never stop creating, please.

ABOUT THE AUTHOR

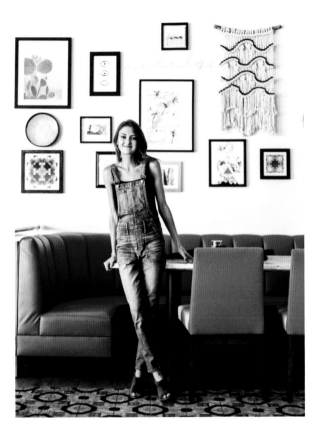

Moriah Sawtelle is an advertising photographer creating and sharing worlds from her base in New York City. A perennial observer, she seeks ordinary moments and shines a light on them in a way that transcends the basic process of living, showing the depth of texture and nuance. If she's not wielding a camera or off pursuing an entrepreneurial idea, you can find her standing in line for coffee with her dog, Hudson.

INDEX